T0144744

BASIC HEALTH
PUBLICATIONS
USER'S GUIDE

TO

NATURAL

THERAPIES FOR

CANCER PREVENTION

AND CONTROL

*Learn How Diet and
Supplements Can
Help Prevent and
Treat Cancer.*

ABRAM HOFFER,
M.D., PH.D., F.R.C.P.(C)

JACK CHALLEM Series Editor

The information contained in this book is based upon the research and personal and professional experiences of the author. It is not intended as a substitute for consulting with your physician or other healthcare provider. Any attempt to diagnose and treat an illness should be done under the direction of a healthcare professional.

The publisher does not advocate the use of any particular healthcare protocol but believes the information in this book should be available to the public. The publisher and author are not responsible for any adverse effects or consequences resulting from the use of the suggestions, preparations, or procedures discussed in this book. Should the reader have any questions concerning the appropriateness of any procedures or preparations mentioned, the author and the publisher strongly suggest consulting a professional healthcare advisor.

Series Editor: Jack Challem
Editor: Karen Anspach
Typesetter: Gary A. Rosenberg
Series Cover Designer: Mike Stromberg

Basic Health Publications User's Guides are published by Basic Health Publications, Inc.

Copyright © 2004 by Abram Hoffer, M.D., Ph.D., F.R.C.P.(C)

ISBN: 978-1-68162-648-2

Printed in the United States of America

10   9   8   7   6   5   4   3   2   1

CONTENTS

ACKNOWLEDGMENTS

I wish to thank the publishing and editorial team members who brought this book to publication. They include Norman Goldfind (publisher), Jack Challem (series editor), Karen Anspach (copyeditor), Janice Malkotsis and Carol Rosenberg (proofreaders), and Gary Rosenberg (typesetter).

INTRODUCTION

The world's major pandemic disease is not AIDS, tuberculosis, or SARS (severe acute respiratory syndrome); it is cancer. Cancer is a leading cause of death, and hardly a family has not mourned the loss of one or more of their members from cancer. It cuts across both sexes, and all ages, countries, and income classes. Almost 624,000 people in Canada and the United States will die from cancer in 2004. Modern medicine has not yet discovered why it occurs or how to treat it effectively, in spite of its overriding emphasis on science, genetics, and antibiotics, and its enormous expenditure on research and development.

Although the Cancer Prevention Coalition (2002) reports that the incidence of smoking-related cancer in men has declined markedly, there has been a major increase in the incidence of predominantly nonsmoking-related cancers in men and women, and also in the incidence of childhood cancers. The National Cancer Institute and American Cancer Society repeatedly misled the public by their assurances of major progress in the war against cancer for over two decades. They completely reversed themselves in May 2002, and admitted that the incidence of cancer is expected to double by 2050.

Current Standard Cancer Treatments

The current three primary treatments for cancer are surgery, radiation, and chemotherapy. Each treatment is serviced by an army of specialists and sub-specialists and supported by the medical literature, our medical institutions, and tons of money. Yet the increase in the ravages of cancer have not been stopped, and the result of the treatments are almost if not as bad as the disease. The impact of the side effects of treatment on the patient's quality of life is too high, the cost of treatment is prohibitive, and the therapeutic results are so dismal that it has been argued that many patients would be better off if they avoided all treatment. Most oncologists (cancer doctors) agree that these three treatment methods have exhausted their potential. They are now placing their hopes on the relatively new research areas that use monoclonal antibodies (a pure type of antibody produced by a single cell), vaccines, anti-angiogenesis drugs (drugs that halt the development of blood vessels), and tyrosine kinase inhibitors (a new group of cancer therapy agents) to fight cancer.

The Need for Alternative Treatment Methods

Because of traditional medicine's lack of success in cancer treatment, alternative and natural cancer therapies have been used for several decades by a few clinicians outside of the vast cancer industry. Their results and conclusions are systematically disregarded or derided, even though there are many case studies published in the medical and alternative literature. Medical progress depends upon the individual efforts of those few dedicated physicians motivated by the need to have better treatment and who are willing to move outside of traditional boundaries; however, the findings of these researchers are ignored. The reason is that our current accepted medical practices rely solely on patented drug therapies and exclude all natural products.

Unfortunately, the potential for further advances in current traditional cancer treatments are limited. Modern surgery is remarkable but probably cannot progress much more, and improvement in radiation treatments and its therapeutic effects will be slow. Chemotherapy works on the principal that it kills the cancer cells but is somewhat less toxic to normal cells. The rate of improvement in chemotherapy is very low. Chemotherapy depends on very expensive drugs controlled by the drug companies.

The cancer establishment demands that proof of research results be based on prospective double-blind, randomized clinical studies. This type of research requires that the method used to analyze data and determine results is described in advance (prospective), that researchers and patients don't know which patients get the "real" treatment and which get a placebo (double blind), and that the variables in the study are applied randomly (randomized). These studies are very costly and usually aren't feasible for clinicians who work outside of institutions funded by other sources, such as drug companies. But such tests are demanded before the possibility will be accepted that nontraditional "outside of the box" biological treatments have value. In my opinion, the present requirements bar is too high and needs to be replaced by the plausibility factor. This means that as the number of good clinical studies (in which a patient is directly observed) increases and are reported, it becomes more and more plausible that natural substances are helpful. When this new, more realistic bar is accepted, there will be a major increase in research to establish the merits of complementary medicine.

The Cancer Prevention Coalition report provides a wide-ranging description of many of the reasons why so little progress has been made in the area of cancer research. It recommends that the role of integrated and holistic medical practice be encouraged. The report states:

> With the growing trend towards pluralism and dialogue, major changes are developing in the understanding and practice of health care. Key is the emergence of integrated and holistic medicine, which poses a powerful challenge to conventional modern high-tech medical practice in industrialized nations, apart from providing low cost care in lesser-developed countries. This challenge has been reinforced by the belated recognition of the ineffectiveness, danger and inflationary impact of a wide range of medical interventions, such as

hormone replacement therapy, and surgery for osteoarthritis of the knee. Not surprisingly, it is estimated that some 40 percent of all Americans are now making many million more visits to integrated and holistic health care providers than to primary care physicians.

Integrated practitioners have clearly established themselves as teachers, rather than just treaters. As such, integrated and holistic practitioners, institutions, and organizations should be mobilized to play a lead role in the STOP CANCER Campaign, and one which could attract larger grass roots support than any other group. They could do this by shifting the current near exclusive emphasis on cancer treatment to at least equal emphasis on primary prevention, and providing the public with information on unknowing exposures to a wide range of avoidable causes of cancer, including carcinogenic prescription drugs, high dose ionizing medical procedures, and carcinogenic ingredient and contaminants in food and other consumer products, besides the importance of healthy and holistic lifestyle practices.

This report could have added orthomolecular medicine as an area that should be integrated and studied, but this term is not well known in medicine and its practices are even less known. Orthomolecular medicine is the practice of preventing and treating biochemical abnormalities, and treating their resulting diseases, through supplementation with optimal amounts of vitamins, amino acids, and other substances naturally found in the body. This is the main reason I have written this book. Its role is to teach, to explain, and to encourage physicians and healers in general and the public at large that there is promise in using natural therapies fortified with optimum, often large, doses of needed nutrients. The plausibility is great that these therapies improve treatment outcome and disease prevention.

Orthomolecular Medicine and Plausibility

Orthomolecular medicine is based on the use of optimum doses of nutrients. The optimum dose range is enormous. These large doses have been called "megadoses," but this term has no accurate meaning, because it varies tremendously depending upon the nutrient and illness. It can mean 3,000 milligrams (mg) of niacin daily when the recommended daily dose to prevent pellagra is about 10 mg, or it can mean 1,000 micrograms (1 mg) of injected vitamin B_{12} when the amount needed to protect against pernicious anemia is 1 microgram (mcg).

In this book, you'll learn about the plausibility that orthomolecular therapy will prolong life and improve its quality when combined with standard-cancer therapy. You'll examine vitamins and minerals and learn how they have been combined to promote improvement in the treatment of cancer. These nutrients are natural components of foods, but they are also available as supplements. A large number of studies show that foods rich in these nutrients prevent cancer. A few studies show that large doses of supplements increase the response rate of treatment when they are combined with standard therapy, and studies are beginning to show that the use of supplements will decrease the incidence of cancer. It is plausible that if they are useful in treatment, they will also be useful in prevention.

CHAPTER 1

ORTHOMOLECULAR MEDICINE'S FOUNDATIONS IN RESEARCH

O rthomolecular medicine was developed by a number of leading researchers studying the relationship of health and disease with nutrition. Many of these researchers are well-known scientists who are recognized and well respected in other specific areas of science, and all believed in the validity of this area of medical research. A brief review of these pioneers and their research will help in understanding the plausibility of orthomolecular medicine.

Dr. Irwin Stone and Early Evidence of High-Dosage Treatment Benefits

Soon after pure vitamin C became available, physicians explored its therapeutic value for a large number of diseases. A few clinical studies showed that adding this vitamin to the treatment of cancer cases improved the patient's prognosis. Dr. Fred Klenner started using huge doses of vitamin C about fifty years ago, and reported that in some cases the results were quite remarkable. These early studies were reviewed by Irwin Stone in his 1972 book, *The Healing Factor.*

Dr. Stone became more directly involved when he interested Dr. Linus Pauling in large dose vitamin treatment. At that time Dr. Pauling was excited about Dr. Klenner's and my use of large amounts of vitamin B_3 for the treatment of schizophrenia. Stone called these large amounts "megadoses." At the meeting where I first met Dr. Pauling and Dr. Stone, Dr. Pauling, at the end of his lecture, remarked that he hoped he could live another twenty-five years, since the advances in science were so exciting. Stone sent him a letter telling him about his research with vitamin C and predicted that if Pauling were to take it himself he would gain the extra years and more. Pauling began to take 3 grams of vitamin C daily. To his delight, he discovered that the frequent colds he had suffered previously no longer troubled him. His book *Vitamin C and the Common Cold* became a very controversial bestseller, and vitamin C sales increased dramatically.

Dr. Linus Pauling and Vitamin C Megadoses for Cancer

A few years later, at a meeting of the newly opened Ben May Institute, Pauling suggested that megadoses of vitamin C might even be helpful in dealing with cancer. The suggestion aroused the ire of Dr. Victor Herbert, a well-known hematologist and nutrition scientist, who became his most powerful critic. Herbert challenged Pauling to present the evidence for his statement. Motivated by this criticism, Pauling reviewed the published literature, and he concluded that there was sufficient evidence to make this idea plausible.

Pauling started a series of studies with Dr. Ewan Cameron, a surgeon in Scotland. They began large-scale therapeutic trials using vitamin C, starting with intravenous doses and later continuing with oral doses. Their book *Cancer and Vitamin C*, published in 1979, describes the impressive results. Cameron and Pauling did not attack the use of standard therapy. In fact, they criticized those who did, writing, "Such a self serving approach is clearly ludicrous; it deliberately ignores the established fact that conventional treatments, based on either scientific fact or empirical discoveries, can cure at least one third of all cancer patients, essentially controlling their disease to such an extent as to give them normal life expectancy. The real objective is to see whether this successful fraction can be even marginally increased by the correct use of all therapeutic resources." Pauling added in his con-

Ascorbate
Another name for vitamin C, which is also called ascorbic acid.

clusion that supplemental ascorbate had a great potential for doing that, when used correctly alongside conventional methods of treating cancer.

The Mayo Clinic Cancer Controversy

The cancer establishment found Pauling's conclusion distasteful and wrong. They looked upon it as a major criticism, ignoring his hope that they continue what they were doing but examine whether the addition of vitamin C might make their results even better. Pauling's enormous status as a two-time Nobel Prize winner meant he could not be ignored, but he was derided by the medical community. It was even suggested his views were the result of early senility. He had committed two serious sins against established medical theory: he supported our use of vitamin B_3 in large doses for treating psychiatric patients, and reinforced the conclusion of a few earlier physicians that megadoses of vitamin C would be helpful for the common cold and flu and, even worse, for the treatment of cancer.

The controversy reached its zenith after the Mayo Clinic published their first report on the treatment of patients with colorectal cancer and concluded that they were unable to corroborate the Cameron and Pauling studies. Although the Clinic had assured Dr. Pauling that they would accurately repeat the conditions of the earlier Cameron and Pauling studies, their work did not duplicate the earlier research methodologies. This controversy is described by Zelek S. Herman, a colleague of Pauling's, in our book *Vitamin C and Cancer: Discovery, Recovery, Controversy*. The controversy and the attitude of the National Cancer Institute are reviewed very carefully and methodically in John Hoffer's contribution to a special workshop on vitamin C and cancer therapy that he chaired at McGill University in Montreal (May 31–June 1, 1999). He wrote, "Looking back on this history, it is difficult to comprehend the cynical disrespect for Cameron and Pauling implicit in the NCI's rejection of their data. The NCI had only to agree 'something happened' at Vale of Leven to be scientifically required from any perspective to acknowledge the need for further investigation. Yet they refused to do so until prodded into it, and when they finally did proceed, the studies were carried out and interpreted with a hostile bias that stacked the odds against a comprehensive, fair evaluation."

The McGill Workshop: Vitamin C as Cancer Therapy

I participated in the McGill workshop from May 31 to June 1, 1999, chaired by John Hoffer, which brought scientists together to consider the state of vitamin C as a therapeutic agent in the treatment of cancer. The participants gave the topic much thought long before we met, and this was reflected in the papers presented and in the free-for-all discussions that followed. Hoffer, Tamayo, and Richardson (2000), three scientists directly involved in the current research, opened the conference with an overview. They pointed out that, "Among the unconventional cancer therapies, high dose vitamin C therapy is the most rigorously studied, most biologically plausible, and most controversial. Both the United States Congress OTA Report, 'Unconventional Cancer Treatments' (1990) and the task force on alternative therapies formed by the Canadian Breast Cancer Research Initiative (1996) concluded that the limited pre-clinical and clinical evidence indicates that vitamin C has potential as an anticancer agent."

John Hoffer (1993, 2000) reviewed the conflict that raged between Linus Pauling and the Mayo group. Linus was very critical of the Mayo group. He said they had not held to their promise to him that they would repeat the earlier Cameron and Pauling studies in every detail, although they claimed they had. He did not deny that the Mayo studies showed no effect, but he did deny them the right to claim that this scientifically negated the whole concept of the original study.

I summarized my data describing the use of high-dosage vitamin C on cancer patients by citing thirty-two ten-year recovery patients out of the first 134 cancer patients I had worked with in my study, a very high success rate. I provided a few case histories to illustrate the results I was getting. Riordan and Riordan (2000) treated their cancer patients with large doses of intravenous sodium ascorbate. They found that high blood levels achieved by intravenous vitamin are cytotoxic, or poisonous, to cancer cells.

A recent report from the Department of Obstetrics and Gynecology, Summa Health System confirmed vitamin C's cytotoxic properties on cancer cells, causing both apoptosis and necrosis (forms of cell death). The toxic effect of vitamin C on cancer cells is enhanced by the addition of alpha lipoic acid, a powerful antioxidant. A few case histories were provided to illustrate the recoveries achieved with this advanced technique.

Antioxidant
A substance that combines with free radicals (unstable atoms or molecules) or other free-radical-producing chemicals to prevent abnormal oxidation or destructive reactions caused by stress, light, or metabolic processes in cells.

The consensus of the meeting was that it is plausible that vitamin C used in therapeutic large doses is helpful in the treatment of cancer and that more clinical studies are warranted. This conclusion should be important to all physicians who treat cancer.

CHAPTER 2

THE START OF ORTHOMOLECULAR MEDICINE

Leading gas companies here (New York) say the Edison's invention has no appreciable effect on gas stocks in this city, and if there is anything of practical value in it, a slight reduction in price may be caused, but it cannot supersede gas for general lighting purposes. They say they have been kept well informed concerning all the recent discoveries in electricity both here and in Europe, and are very skeptical about the promised electrical millennium which is to abolish gas.

—December 24, 1879, from the *Globe and Mail* (Toronto, October 21, 2003)

It is unfortunately the case that traditional medicine follows other branches of science and invention in ignoring or scorning many important discoveries until long after their initial introduction. In 1968, Linus Pauling published his paper, "Orthomolecular Psychiatry, in Science," and provided a scientific, theoretical, and practical basis for the concepts of orthomolecular medicine. He defined orthomolecular medicine "for the preservation of good health and the treatment of disease by varying the concentrations in the body of substances that are normally present in the body and are required for health." This definition referred to a new concept, or paradigm, in medicine with respect to the use of supplements for treating disease. The older and still highly respected paradigm is called "vitamins as prevention." This concept supports the use of very small doses of a few vitamins

Paradigm
A term used in science to describe a general concept or viewpoint under which a discipline, subdiscipline, or theory is developed.

needed to prevent the occurrence of a few deficiency diseases such as pellagra. With the vitamins-as-prevention paradigm, vitamin supplements are not needed except for preventing these diseases, and megadoses are never required.

Pellagra
A disease caused by a deficiency of niacin (nicotinic acid). Symptoms include gastrointestinal problems, diarrhea, dermatitis, mental disorders, and ultimately death.

The new paradigm, which is currently gaining favor, called "vitamins as treatment," originated with our findings in 1955 that 3 grams of niacin per day lowered cholesterol levels. Three grams of niacin is a megadose, and hypercholesterolemia (high cholesterol) is not a vitamin-deficiency disease. Pauling's definition allowed for optimum doses, which might range from very small to very large, to be used as treatment for all types of diseases.

My First Cancer Patient

I became interested in cancer when a psychotic patient with terminal cancer of the lung survived his prognosis by twenty-eight months. It was 1960, and at the time, I was searching for a biochemical unique to patients with schizophrenia. We discovered a substance in the urine that we called the "mauve factor," as it stained mauve color on the paper chromatograms. For comparison, we also analyzed the urine of normal subjects and patients suffering very severe stress, such as terminal cancer. Most of the eight cancer patients I tested excreted this substance. A psychotic, delirious seventy-five-year-old man with terminal lung cancer was admitted to the psychiatric ward. He had been treated with cobalt bomb radiation. The cancer clinic concluded that he could not live more than a month or two. I tested his urine and found he

Chromatography
Analyzes complex mixtures, such as urine, by separating them into the chemicals from which they are made. A paper chromatogram charts the different components in the mixture.

excreted huge quantities of the mauve factor.

By then we knew from our previous therapeutic trials that psychiatric patients who excreted the mauve factor responded very well to treatment with large doses of vitamin B_3 (niacin or niacinamide). I suggested to his resident that he start him on 3 grams of niacin daily. He was started on this dosage on a Friday, and by the following Monday, he was mentally normal. I was interested in seeing what the long-term effect of the vitamin would be on his psychiatric state, so I offered to provide both the niacin and vitamin C to him for free if he would come to my office each month to obtain it. A year later, I was surprised when the cancer clinic informed me that they could no longer see any lesion in his lung. On each of his visits every three months, they had seen a reduction in the size of his cancer. He died twenty-eight months after I started him on the vitamin. I thought the niacin might be the most important factor in the remission of the cancer since it was (and still is) my favorite vitamin. I had added vitamin C only because I did so routinely for my schizophrenic patients, but the exciting work of Cameron and Pauling suggested that the vitamin C was the more important single remission factor.

Cobalt Bomb Radiation
The popular name of the original radiation therapy that used the cobalt-60 radioactive isotope. It is the grandfather of the radiation therapy units now used in modern cancer facilities.

Recovery of a Patient from Cancer of the Pancreas

In 1976 I moved to Victoria, British Columbia. By this time, I was well known because of my interest in the use of vitamins. In July 1978, A.S., born in 1919, was referred to me with cancer of the pancreas. She died in 1999.

A.S.'s death is not remarkable; many people die in their eighties. Most cancer patients, however, die within five years, and hardly any cases of cancer of the pancreas survive even one year. What is remarkable is that she did not die twenty-two years earlier, when she was first referred to me. She disobeyed the Cancer Clinic's prediction that she would be dead within three to six months. She read Norman Cousins' book *Anatomy of an Illness*, and inspired by this remarkable account of his recovery with large doses of vitamin C and laughter, she took large doses of vitamin C.

In May 1978 she had become jaundiced. A laparotomy (a surgical incision through the abdominal wall) was performed, which revealed complete obstruction of the common bile duct by a six-centimeter diameter hard mass in the head of the pancreas. This was judged to be a carcinoma (cancer). The associated lymph glands were clear and no distant metastases (tumors) were detected, so it appeared the cancer had not spread. Since it was felt that biopsy would risk spreading the tumor, no biopsy was taken. A cholecystojejunostomy was performed to open the channel between the gallbladder and the jejunum (a section of the small intestine).

Jaundice
Yellowing of the skin and whites of the eyes caused by an interruption in the flow of bile through the body. Bile is a digestive juice produced by the liver.

A.S. was referred to me for evaluation and further treatment. I advised her referring doctor to increase her vitamin C intake as much as possible, and added the rest of the program. Within a few months, she was taking 40 grams of vitamin C daily. I also told her to take 500 mg of niacinamide three times a day, and 220 mg of zinc sulfate once a day, and advised her to follow a high vegetable and fruit, low meat diet that excluded junk food. She adhered to this regimen for five years.

After the first five years, she took about 5 grams of ascorbic acid crystals, a pure form of vitamin C, along with 500 mg of niacinamide and an unspecified amount of vitamin E every day.

Dr. D. Kanofsky interviewed her for Linus Pauling. He found that although she was given three months to live at the time of her May 1978 operation, she still led an active life eleven years later. There had been no recurrence of any cancer. An abdominal sonogram (also called an ultrasound) in June 1978 showed a predominately translucent area in the porta hepatis area of the liver, which was judged to be a tumor. This mass was no longer seen in the abdominal CT scan performed in January 1979, or in subsequent CT scans.

CT Scan (Computed Tomography Scan)

A computerized series of low-intensity X rays that produce detailed cross-sectional images of the body and can reveal disease or abnormalities in tissue and bone.

A.S. worked in a bookstore. She was so happy with her recovery that she told anyone who would listen to her about it. Five months after I saw her for the second time, she called me at home on a Sunday evening. She was very excited and told me that she had just two successive CT scans. The first one did not show any tumor. The radiologist could not believe this was true and repeated it.

The following year about five more patients came to see me, and over the next ten years I saw about 135 patients. In almost every case, they found it difficult to find a physician who would refer them to me because I am a clinical psychiatrist. One reason was that since the patients did not have any psychiatric problems, it was difficult to refer them to a psychiatrist. The more important reason, however, was that they did not believe vitamins would play any useful function, and that it would be a waste of time or might interfere with chemotherapy. Many doctors tried assiduously to persuade their patients not to come, and many patients changed doctors so they could see me. By the end of 2003, about 1,300 cancer patients had been referred to me.

The First Forty Patients and the Plausibility of High-Dosage Therapy

After I had seen around forty patients, I began to suspect that the patients who were following their program were living longer and had a better quality of life. I followed up every patient I had seen and compared the outcome of the patients who followed the program against those who did not or could not follow it, using the number of months they remained alive from the time they were first seen until the day they died as the outcome measure. A smaller number of patients did not follow the program because their families would not support them, or because their family doctors made fun of them, or because they died before they could remain on the program for at least two months. Obviously, a treatment lasting only a few weeks would not be a proper test of the efficacy of the program. I, therefore, divided my patients into two groups: those who followed the program at least two months, and those who did not. The difference was clinically significant.

The Hoffer-Pauling Reports

Several years later, Dr. Pauling and I participated in a seminar honoring Dr. Arthur Sackler at Woods Hole, Massachusetts. He encouraged me to expand my follow-up series on my cancer patients, and asked me if I intended to publish my findings. I replied that I hadn't intended to publish because I didn't think I could find a publisher, but Dr. Pauling told me that if I did the follow-up work, he would help me find one. I agreed.

I still had not extended my follow-up work when I heard from Pauling two years later, asking me how I was getting along. That was my final motivation. I reviewed the files of every one of the first 134 patients I had seen, and Pauling and I examined the resulting data. We concluded that 80 percent of the patients who followed the regimen had a probable survival time sixteen times that of the thirty-one control patients. The average survival time for the control patient was 5.7 months, which is close to the survival times of ambulatory terminal cancer patients (Hoffer and Pauling, 1990). By the end of 1993, I had seen 636 patients. Of these patients, 518 followed the regimen treatment and 118 were not on the treatment.

The actual survival times for this larger group of patients were remarkably close to the estimated survivals by Linus Pauling using the Hardin Jones statistical method.

My follow-up was not a prospective double-blind, randomized therapeutic trial, or a research trial. It was an analysis of many patients treated for a variety of problems, who had been referred to me by their family doctors, surgeons, or oncologists. I could not have done this type of formal study on this patient group even though I am thoroughly familiar with the design of the double-blind trial, having directed double-blind therapeutic trials in 1952 to investigate the therapeutic properties of vitamin B_3 in the treatment of schizophrenia when I was director of psychiatric research for the Province of Saskatchewan.

Since I did not have a randomized control for my patient group, the best I could do was to compare the outcome of the treatment group against the smaller group who did not remain on the program for at least two months. Although this was not a randomized controlled study, the selection of patients into each group was more or less random and depended upon a large number of factors over which I had no control. This non-randomized control group had the same outcome in general as that found in ambulatory terminal cancer patients. The treated group had a much better prognosis.

CHAPTER 3

Nutrition, Diet, and Vitamins in the Orthomolecular Program

Orthomolecular medicine is often labeled as an alternative or complementary medical practice by traditional practitioners. Such labeling attempts to ignore the fact that orthomolecular medicine was established by respected, experienced research scientists, and is recognized and practiced by many medical doctors who have seen the value of its theories. Orthomolecular medicine does not undermine current medical practices; it provides additional preventive and treatment options to patients based on sound nutritional and biological principles. The basis of these principles is founded on nutrition, diet, and the positive intake of supplements that can assist the body in fighting disease. This chapter describes the importance of these nutritional elements, and how vitamins and minerals can help combat diseases such as cancer.

The Importance of Nutrition and Diet

All organisms live in a very intimate relationship with their environment. The external environment provides the food supply and nutrients essential for life, directly influencing the organism's internal environment and health. This is a complex interrelationship that is subject to continual fluctuations. Over evolutionary time, all species have had to adapt their internal systems to survive these external changes and maintain health. Of all the external influences, there is nothing more important than good nutrition.

We have been adapted to the Stone-Age diet that early humans ate for over a million years. Essentially, this diet excludes all the members of the grass family except in very small quantities. It excludes all sugars except for small amounts of honey, and it excludes dairy products, because these foods were rarely if ever available. The modern refinements to our diet be-gan to develop about 9,000 years ago with the dawn of agriculture, and are therefore relatively new introductions to the human diet. These dietary changes have accelerated at a remarkable rate over the past 100 years. About fifty years ago, around 15 percent of the food consumed in Canada was processed in some manner. Today, this figure is close to 85 percent. For more information on this topic, see my book *Hoffer's Laws of Natural Nutrition: A Guide to Eating Well for Pure Health* (1996).

Processed Foods
Foods that have been subjected to special processes to give them certain characteristics or to make them stay fresh longer. To do this, chemicals, refined sugar, salt, and other flavor enhancers are added. Foods lose much of their original enzymes and nutrients as a result.

Many people think that they can eat a poor diet, high in processed and fast foods, as long as they take supplements such as vitamins. Although supplements can repair some of the consequences of poor nutrition to a remarkable degree, they cannot by themselves replace the need for a proper diet. Supplements should be added after the diet has been corrected. Not every one of the fifteen known vitamins needs to be supplemented, but it is important that none is lacking in a proper diet and supplementation program.

Food—What to Eat

The relationship between food and cancer is well established. Diets rich in vegetables and fruit decrease the incidence of cancer. The connection between cancer and diets high or low in protein, fat, or carbohydrates is still very controversial. I think this is due to the individuality of people—our needs are not the same. Some people may need vegetarian diets; others may need high-protein diets. The basis of the Kelly treatment, a metabolic cancer-cure diet, depends upon first determining which particular diet should be followed by each individual. I advise my patients to increase their intake of fruit, vegetables, and fish and to sharply limit their intake of junk foods. Junk food is any food or preparation that contains added free sugars. Sugar increases the metabolic burden on the body, which is not good for cancer patients. I also ask patients to eliminate any foods they know they are allergic to, on the principle that their immune system should be dealing with their cancer as much as possible and not have the additional burden of dealing with allergic foods.

Finally, everyone's diet should be palatable. Enjoyment of food is a very important contributor to good health. A diet that is bland or repulsive will certainly not make it easier for cancer patients, who already have too much pressure on them.

About Vitamins

Vitamins are organic compounds that catalyze reactions in the body. They are needed in very small amounts to prevent the occurrence of vitamin deficiency diseases. Diets that are deficient in very small amounts of vitamin C, vitamin B_3, vitamin D_3, and thiamine will cause diseases such as scurvy, pellagra, rickets, and beriberi. This original definition of vitamins was very helpful when scientists were first identifying vitamins to isolate them through the diseases caused by their deficiencies.

A vitamin is a compound that our bodies cannot make on their own. A good example is vitamin C, which is not a vitamin for most animals who can make all they need. Vitamin C cannot be made by humans or our closest relatives the monkeys and apes, or by the guinea pig. We lost the ability to manufacture vitamin C millions of years ago. Pauling showed how this inability could have been advantageous, if we had continued to live on foods that were rich in vitamin C.

Vitamin Supplements—How Much?

The daily requirements that have been enshrined by government health agencies are based on an average, normal, healthy person. They are of no value for people under stress, or those who are sick, addicted, pregnant, or nursing. They do not take into account differences in people's height, weight, and so on. These officially sanctioned daily requirements may have some value for less than half of the population. Optimal daily requirements have not yet been determined for those suffering from different diseases. Current laboratory tests are not very useful, since blood values do not tell us much about the state of health within the body's cells. For example, many patients become well when they are given 1 mg injections of vitamin B_{12}, even though their blood levels of B_{12} are within the normal range. The clinical findings and the response of the patient to supplementation is a much superior determinant to any of the tests.

When it comes to water-soluble vitamins, I follow the rule that it is better for the body to have more rather than less because the surplus is easily excreted and does no harm. This rule has to be applied more carefully with the few fat-soluble vitamins, but even with these vitamins, the toxicity danger has been grossly exaggerated.

I practice the opposite rule when it comes to vitamin supplementation than I do for drugs. I think that one should use slightly less drugs than what has been recommended by the drug companies, because less is less dangerous than more. The special issue of the *Journal of Orthomolecular Medicine* (2003) contains a complete description of the safety and lack of toxicity of the main orthomolecular vitamins.

Vitamins-as-Prevention Paradigm

According to traditional medical belief, vitamins are needed only to avoid vitamin deficiency diseases and in very small amounts. These theories have been enshrined into official recommendations by governments who established average daily requirements. Rigid adherence to this concept of supplementation created many problems, because it meant that vitamins were not needed if these deficiency diseases were not present. It also meant that large doses of vitamins were never indicated. As mentioned earlier, this belief is known as the "vitamins-as-prevention" paradigm. Even when this paradigm served at its best, there was already evidence that it was faulty, because many chronic or deficiency diseases take many years to reveal themselves. This is discussed by Robert P. Heaney, who describes diseases such as rickets as "short-latency deficiency disease" and diseases such as cancer as "long-latency deficiency diseases." The vitamins-as-prevention paradigm offers protection only against short-latency deficiency diseases.

Early pellagrologists (doctors treating pellagra) in the United States found that niacin given in vitamin (small) doses cured the disease, unless it was chronic and had been present for a long time. Chronic patients had to be given as much as 600 mg of niacin daily, which was considered a huge dose in 1935. These chronic patients required much larger doses of niacin than were needed to prevent pellagra from first occurring and to prevent pellagra from reoccurring.

Vitamins-as-Treatment Paradigm

The "vitamins-as-treatment" paradigm's roots go back to the 1940s, when four doctors began to use large doses of vitamins to treat disease. Drs. Evan Shute and Wilfred Shute in Ontario used vitamin E to treat heart disease and accelerate burn healing, Dr. Fred Klenner in North Carolina used vitamin C for a large variety of severe infectious diseases and multiple sclerosis, and Dr. William Kaufman in New York used niacinamide to treat arthritis. Their findings were ignored and discounted by the medical community. My colleagues' and my report on the cholesterol-lowering action of niacin in 1955 alerted a few physicians, however. Today, niacin is the gold standard for lowering cholesterol and triglyceride levels, elevating high-density lipoprotein cholesterol levels (the "good" cholesterol), and decreasing deaths from cardiovascular disease.

We were all using vitamins in large doses to treat

conditions not known to be vitamin-deficiency diseases. This new paradigm is gradually moving into traditional medicine. Bruce Ames and associates expanded upon Pauling's work, showing that high-dose vitamin therapy is needed to stimulate variant enzymes that have a decreased coenzymes binding affinity. Variant enzymes (defective enzymes that have lost some of their ability to perform their specific functions) do not have the same ability to bind (link to) vitamins as the original enzymes, and it takes a lot more to force the vitamin onto the enzyme. About fifty human genetic diseases are known to be due to these defective enzymes, and many more will be discovered.

Enzymes
Naturally occurring proteins in the human body that help the body's chemistry work. Coenzymes are small molecules that act as enzyme activators or catalysts.

I defined diseases that require large doses of vitamins to be treated as "vitamin-dependent" diseases. Arthritics or schizophrenic patients who get well when they are given large doses of niacin are examples of patients suffering from vitamin dependencies. I concluded this from observing a natural experiment that should never be done again. In World War II, over 2,000 Canadian soldiers were sent to protect Hong Kong. They were promptly captured and incarcerated for forty-four months in prisoner of war camps, along with soldiers from the United States and England. These places were so awful and so stressful that up to one-third of the soldiers died. The soldiers saved from the camps remained ill afterward, and had a very high morbidity and death rate from cardiovascular, neurological, and psychiatric diseases. The exceptions who recovered were a few who came under my care and were placed on high doses of niacin. I estimated that one year in the camps aged my patients at least four years. The soldiers who survived forty-four months came home about fifteen years older. I concluded that the long exposure to nutritional deficiencies, infections, and cruelty had altered their body chemistry to the point that that they could no longer remain well on the usual vitamin doses. They needed 3 grams or more of vitamin B_3 daily, for the remainder of their lives. Chronic deficiency had become chronic dependency.

Recently, R.P. Heaney (2003) came to the same conclusions from a series of elegant studies on vitamin D, calcium, and folic acid. He called this condition long-latency deficiency disease (LLDD). He wrote:

> Discerning the full role of nutrition in long-latency, multifactorial disorders is probably the principal challenge facing nutritional science today. The first component of this challenge is to recognize that inadequate intakes of specific nutrients may produce more than one disease, may produce diseases by more than one mechanism, and may require several years for the consequent morbidity to be sufficiently evident to be clinically recognizable as "disease." Because the intakes required to prevent many of the long-latency disorders are higher than those required to prevent the respective index disease, recommendations based solely on preventing the index disease are no longer biologically defensible.

Deficiency of niacin is an excellent example of Dr. Healy's description. A short exposure to insufficient niacin causes pellagra. This is the index disease, which is easily treated with very small doses of vitamin B_3. Long exposure to the deficient state creates a condition in which the disease is no longer responsive to these small doses, and leads to a variety of symptoms, including abnormalities of blood lipids and probably cardiovascular and cerebrovascular disease, arthritis, and early aging.

A special issue of the *Journal of Orthomolecular Medicine* entitled "The Safety and Efficacy of Vitamins" is available for further reading on this topic. We published this special issue to answer the many patently absurd, erroneous, or exaggerated claims made about vitamins by members of the vitamins-as-prevention school, and published widely by the press. The issue describes the following vitamins and their relationship to cancer: vitamin A (and beta-carotene), vitamin B$_3$, vitamin B$_6$, folic acid, vitamin C, vitamin D, and vitamin E. This is a very valuable issue and should be read to supplement this book. It will reassure you about the remarkable safety of vitamins when they are used as therapy.

Vitamin Cocktails

In 1952, we began to use two vitamins for treating schizophrenia, vitamins B$_3$ and C. In our double-blind, controlled studies, we were forced to omit the vitamin C, because our design consultant advised that it would be too complicated to work with two nutrients. (This is one of the disadvantages of this methodology.) However, we almost always used it thereafter. Later, as I became more familiar with other members of the B vitamin family, I began to add them to the program. The most common was the B-complex preparation, which contained almost all the B vitamins, including small amounts of folic acid and vitamin B$_{12}$.

I was already using a vitamin cocktail when I began to treat patients with cancer. The vitamins described in this book are all part of this cocktail approach. It turned out that, in fact, there is a major advantage in using several antioxidants together, because they reinforce one another. In mid-2003, the British Broadcasting Corporation reported on a major dietary supplement study in France and England. More than 13,000 subjects were given small amounts of beta-carotene, vitamin C, vitamin E, and zinc. Over a seven-year period, the incidence of cancer decreased by one-third in those taking the supplements, when compared to the placebo control group.

A recent Cancer Prevention Study II Nutrition Cohort in the United States involving 145,000 subjects found that regular use of multivitamin supplementation started ten years earlier was associated with a reduction in colon cancer risk. A news release from the Multivitamin and Public Health: Exploring the Evidence meeting reported that the daily use of a multivitamin by older adults would lead to more than $1.6 billion in Medicare savings over five years. These potential savings would rise, from reduction in rates of hospitalization for heart attacks and a reduction in admission to hospitals, nursing homes, and home healthcare services. They reported that most Americans do not get optimum amounts of key micronutrients through diet alone, and that daily multivitamins should be taken, that they are safe, cost effective and accessible, and that that evidence supporting these conclusions is very promising. These views are supported by David Heber, M.D., Ph.D., Director, UCLA Center for Human Nutrition, and J. Blumberg, Ph.D., Friedman School of Nutrition Sciences and Policy at Tufts University.

CHAPTER 4

VITAMIN C
(ASCORBIC ACID)

Vitamin C is probably the most widely taken vitamin supplement in the world. It is available as vitamin C (hydrogen ascorbate) and also as a mineral salt with sodium, or calcium or potassium. It can be taken by mouth or by intravenous injection using sodium ascorbate. It is present in fruits and vegetables in very small amounts. Citrus fruits are among the better sources, but the amount of vitamin C present will vary, depending upon the way the fruit is handled between the orchard and the table. Even the most favorable vitamin C–rich diet will not provide optimum health for most people.

The Safety of Vitamin C Supplementation

S. Lawson (2003) wrote a complete account of vitamin C's safety. Vitamin C is safe—it is less toxic than every over-the-counter drug freely available—but there is nothing that is absolutely 100 percent safe, not even drinking water. The safety of any substance must be determined by comparing it against something that everyone recognizes as safe. The acid test of safety is the body count—how many deaths are caused by the substance? Dangerous drugs do kill. Vitamins do not. There have been no deaths reported for vitamin C and no toxicity data on humans. If one could engage in a duel using chemicals as the weapon, and I were to fight such a duel, I would have a bowl of vitamin C in front of me and would take one level teaspoon every few minutes. My opponent would have a bowl of ordinary table salt in front of him, and would match me spoon by spoon. The salt will kill him. The vitamin C will not kill me.

There are both negative and positive side effects

to vitamin C supplementation. The main positive side effect is that it is the most important water-soluble antioxidant available, and totally essential for general health. The main side effect is that it causes loose stools if the dose is high enough. If a laxative is needed, this becomes a positive side effect. If the stools are too loose, it becomes a negative side effect. This side effect varies enormously with each person and with the intensity of any disease present. Dr. Robert Cathcart found that patients who were sick could tolerate a lot more vitamin C before loose stools developed. A person with a severe cold may be able to tolerate very large doses, but will not be able to tolerate that much once the cold is gone. A large enough dosage must be taken for maximum therapeutic effect, however, and the development of loose stools is a good marker or indicator that the therapeutic level has been reached.

The optimum vitamin C dosage may range from 1 gram to 75 grams daily by mouth. Very few people can tolerate the larger amounts, and most will take between 3 and 20 grams daily in divided doses. It is best not to take the entire dose at one time. The body uses vitamin C more efficiently if it is taken after each meal. For cancer patients, I recommend dissolving the daily dosage in juice, storing it in the fridge, and drinking a portion six times over the course of the day. Vitamin C is not stable in pure water as it is oxidized by traces of copper, but this reaction is inhibited in juice. It is important to reach the maximum blood concentration as vitamin C is rapidly excreted. A few patients cannot tolerate the pure vitamin C because of its sour taste and acidity, but they may find the calcium and sodium ascorbate form much more palatable.

Much larger doses of sodium ascorbate can be given intravenously, and as much as 200 grams have been given in this manner over a period of many hours without side effects. Pure ascorbic acid is too acidic and must not be used intravenously. Dr. Klenner used to give patients 50 to 100 grams intravenously over four to six hours for the treatment of cancer. Dr. Hugh Riordan found that these high doses of ascorbic acid killed cancer cells, so it acts as a benign form of chemotherapy. Vitamin C never has a laxative effect when it is taken intravenously.

Mechanism of Action

Vitamin C is intimately involved in so many reactions in the body it would be very surprising if it did not have remarkable antitumor activity. It is a major scavenger of free radicals in the body, which are known to cause cellular damage. In their excellent report, C. Tamayo and M.A. Richardson (2003) listed thirteen ways in which vitamin C might exert its beneficial activity in dealing with cancer. The most important mechanisms will be discovered when vitamin C's real potential is accepted and more funding is devoted to studying its characteristics.

Oncologist's Unreasonable Fear of Vitamin C and Other Antioxidants

In his comprehensive book, *Antioxidants and Cancer,* Ralph Moss concludes, "It is an uncontested fact that synthetic antioxidants do not have a negative impact on radiation and chemotherapy treatment, nor do oncologists fear that they might. Instead synthetic antioxidants preserve the effectiveness of conventional treatments while reducing their harmful side effects. The data also supports the idea that dietary antioxidants protect against harmful side effects without interfering with the cancer killing ability of conventional treatments. And natural antioxidants do this without toxic side effects of their own and at a fraction of the cost of these synthetic agents."

Why do oncologists fear these natural antioxidants, usually vitamin C, but not the xenobiotic antioxidants provided by drug companies? Is it another example of the pervasive negative feeling in the medical com-

Xenobiotic
A chemical compound that does not occur naturally and is foreign to the biological systems exposed to it. This term is often used to refer to human-made chemicals that are resistant to biodegradation and decomposition.

munity about vitamins in general and specifically for vitamin C, the body's most important water-soluble antioxidant? In fact, the College of Physicians and Surgeons of one of Canada's provinces ordered a physician to not prescribe vitamins to any cancer patients receiving or about to receive conventional treatment. One oncologist advised his patient that if he took vitamin C, he would no longer treat him. What is the source of this unreasonable position, this paranoia, when the clinical research evidence is entirely positive and favors the use of these natural antioxidants? According to Moss, it started following ". . . a 1999 polemic by a naturopath, Dan Labriola, and oncologist Robert Livingston in the journal *Oncology.*"

There are no clinical series showing that the patients given both vitamin C and chemotherapy fare worse than those not given this vitamin. On the contrary, all of the published series show just the opposite. I have treated over 1,300 cases with large doses of vitamin C, and most of them also had chemotherapy. I have examined the follow-up data and compared patients taking vitamins and those not taking vitamins, but with otherwise similar treatment, and find that the use of the vitamins heavily favored the prolongation of life. Recently, K.N. Prasad, et al. (1999), after reviewing seventy-one scientific papers, found no evidence that antioxidants interfered with the therapeutic effect of chemotherapy. Simone (1992) came to the same conclusion even earlier.

The article in *Oncology* by Labriola et al. (1999) that reinforced the negative beliefs of the medical profession concluded that vitamin C may prevent the therapeutic effect of chemotherapy if given concurrently, and recommended that antioxidants be withheld until after chemotherapy is completed. He based his conclusion on one case that suggested this had occurred, and upon a hypothetical examination of the role of free radicals and antioxidants on the action of chemotherapy on cancer cells. His report elicited two rebuttals: Reilly (2001) and Gignac (2000).

Drs. Labriola and Livingston did not consider the

following points. What is the therapeutic value of chemotherapy, even without the addition of any antioxidants? Even within the field of traditional oncology, there is a debate over whether chemotherapy has any merit, except for a small number of cancers, Moss (2000). Before one can claim that a treatment has been inhibited, there must be pretty good evidence that the treatment has merit to begin with. Although chemotherapy is accepted as a conventional treatment, the scientific evidence is not as solid as one would like. It is possible (we do not know the probability) that the reverse is true, and that chemotherapy interferes with the therapeutic value of the antioxidants. Almost all the studies testing large doses of vitamin C yielded positive results, while there is no such unanimity with respect to chemotherapy. Significantly, these studies use the word "may," not "will." There is a difference between possibility and probability, even though most people do not distinguish between these two. Theoretically anything is possible, and it is certainly possible that taking vitamin C might prevent the toxic but beneficial effect of chemotherapy. The important statistic is probability. What is the probability that patients receiving vitamin C during their chemotherapy will not fare as well as those who do not? We can only assume from the literature reviewed that the real probability must be extremely low. As I have pointed out earlier, I have seen no evidence that adding vitamin C inhibits the therapeutic effect of chemotherapy. Just the opposite seems to be the case; patients on my orthomolecular program live substantially longer, and about 40 percent achieved four-year cure rates. Given the attitude of traditional medicine, it is not surprising that *Oncology* accepted this single patient anecdote for publication. I doubt they would have accepted a similar anecdote if it was supportive of the use of vitamin C.

Moss further points out that oncologists have no objection to using xenobiotic antioxidants during chemotherapy. This includes Amifostine, which decreases the toxicity of radiation but is too toxic on its own and is not used; Mesna, a drug used around the world to protect against the toxic side effects of ifosfamide, which damages the urinary system, and Cardiozane, which counters Adriamycin's toxicity. There are more than 500 papers showing the safety of Cardiozane. In one clinical trial using a drug similar to Adriamycin, one-quarter of the patients suffered damage to their hearts. When given Cardiozane concurrently only 7 percent did. Synthetic antioxidants protect against the toxic effect of chemotherapy drugs, but do not increase their therapeutic value. In sharp contrast, natural antioxidants not only protect against the toxic effect of chemotherapy drugs, but also increase their efficacy in destroying cancer cells. Yet, according to many in the medical community, only orthomolecular or natural antioxidants are potentially dangerous.

Recently, Stoute (2003) came to the same conclusion as did Moss. She analyzed forty-four scientific and other articles on the effectiveness of vitamin C in chemotherapy when used alone and with other vitamins. She found that of the forty-four articles, twenty-four were studies that were positive toward the use of vitamin C and other vitamins, twelve were positive reviews, one was neutral, one was negative, two were negative reviews, and four were responses to the latter two. Stoute concluded, ". . . this annotated bibliography of literature on the effectiveness of vitamin C alone or with other vitamins, during chemotherapy confirms conclusions of Prasad and coworkers (1999): 'antioxidants (including vitamin C) do not protect cancer cells against free radical and growth inhibiting effects of standard therapy. On the contrary, they enhance its growth-inhibitory effects on tumor cells, but protect normal cells against its adverse effects.'" Stoute's review included the Tamayo, Richardson report, which references the studies showing the safety of vitamin C.

What are the odds that one anecdotal report on one patient in which it is suggested that vitamin C might be adverse would be adopted so rapidly by the huge oncological and radiological establishments worldwide, while so many positive studies and reviews are ignored? Apparently the odds are pretty good, if you don't like the concept being dismissed and the report appears in an establishment journal.

Drisko, Chapman, and Hunter's very recent (2003) report was included in Stoute's review. This study from University of Kansas Medical School reported that two patients with ovarian cancer were alive and well thirty months later after receiving chemotherapy and large doses of vitamin C orally and intravenously. The authors concluded that the addition of the antioxidants improved the clinical results, and they are conducting larger scale studies. They questioned the concept that antioxidants are contraindicated during most chemotherapy regimens, stating that it was no longer valid. This is the concept on which the antagonism toward vitamin C is based.

Vitamin C provides some protection against radiation skin burns. Two patients who had taken vitamin C wanted reconstructive surgery after they had completed their series of radiation treatments. Normally, plastic surgeons will not do reconstruction work on these patients because their skin is so damaged from the radiation. With these two patients, the skin was not damaged, and they were able to have the surgery.

Another possible effect that vitamin C may provide is that it may protect children who have survived their cancers. According to studies reported by the Professor of Pediatrics at the University of Texas Southwestern Medical Center, nearly half of all child cancer survivors develop significant physical and mental health problems in adulthood. I think it is plausible that vitamin C, which is a good antioxidant, would protect against the free radicals created by the radiation and thus decrease the toxic effects that occur later in life.

Other Current Factoids about Vitamin C

A large number of factoids have circulated—and many still are circulating—in the medical profession about the supposed dangers of vitamin C. These

Factoid
Unverified or invented information that resembles a fact and is believed because it appeared in print.

factoids are based upon unproven hypotheses. There is no clinical data to support any of them, and all actual studies have revealed that they are not true. None of them are supported by any controlled studies. Here is a brief list, but I will not discuss them in detail. Claims were widely circulated by the press that vitamin C causes the following conditions: kidney stones, kidney damage, pernicious anemia, decreased fertility in women, liver damage, iron overload and toxicity, and cancer; that it is dangerous for diabetics because it interferes with glucose tests; that it increases arteriosclerosis in coronary arteries; and shortened Linus Pauling's life (he died at age 94).

Interaction Between Vitamin C and Other Antioxidants

NAD←>NADH
The active enzyme that contains nicotinamide. The NAD←>NADH system is one of the most active oxidation-reduction systems.

I did not use only vitamin C when I started my series in 1978 because I wanted to increase the efficacy of the results by using other antioxidants such as vitamin E succinate, and sometimes beta-carotene, selenium, and vitamin B_3, which in the body is converted to the NAD←>NADH system.

Prasad found that using several antioxidants is preferable, based upon laboratory studies that showed that when vitamin C, vitamin E, and beta-carotene were combined the mixture was always toxic to cancer cells, whereas when they were used individually they were not always toxic. Vitamin C is the most important vitamin in the treatment of cancer, but other nutrients have antitumor properties. The use of multivitamin and multimineral regimens is preferable to the use of any one alone.

CHAPTER 5

VITAMIN B₃

Vitamin B$_3$ is the anti-pellagra vitamin. Adding niacinamide to flour almost eradicated pellagra, a disease that was a major scourge in the Southeast United States until the cause of pellagra was discovered. There are several forms of vitamin B$_3$. All are equivalent as vitamins, but there are differences as well. Niacinamide (also known as nicotinamide) is the one most commonly added to multivitamin preparations because it does not cause vasodilatation or flushing. It has no effect on blood lipid levels, and has not been tested for any protective effect against vascular disease. Niacin (also known as nicotinic acid) acts as a vasodilator when it is first taken. It is the gold standard for lowering cholesterol, triglycerides, and lipoprotein A, and for elevating high-density lipoprotein cholesterol. It also decreases deaths in patients who have already had one coronary. It is available in no-flush forms, which have to be carefully formulated. Inositol niacinate is a combination of two vitamins, inositol and niacin. The niacin is released from this compound so slowly that it does not cause flushing. It also has an effect on lipids, but it is not as effective as niacin. All the forms are equally therapeutic for the arthritides (inflammations of the joints), for healing, and for cancer. When I think circulation should be improved, I prefer niacin as a vasodilator. For my cancer-treatment program, I use 300 mg to 3 grams daily.

Vitamin B$_3$

A water-soluble, coenzyme vitamin that helps the body release energy from proteins, fat, and carbohydrates. It is important for healthy skin, nerves, digestion, and memory.

Proper Vitamin B$_3$ Dosages

The proper vitamin B$_3$ dose depends upon the condition being treated. The vitamin requirement for preventing pellagra is very small. The therapeutic dose to treat existing pellagra depends on how long the condition has been present, and will vary from the usual low dose to 600 mg daily.

The niacin dose for lowering cholesterol is 3 to 9 grams daily; for treating schizophrenia, it is 3 to 12 grams daily; and for treating arthritis, it is 500 mg to 3 grams daily. For most other conditions, less than 3 grams daily are needed. The dose of niacinamide is usually 3 grams daily or less, but more is required for treating schizophrenia, and up to 9 grams per day is needed for reinforcing the therapeutic effect of radiation in treating some cancers. The dose of inositol niacinate is in the same range. These are very rough guidelines only. In each case, the patient's response will determine their optimum dose.

Side Effects of Vitamin B$_3$

The main side effect of niacin is the initial flush. This starts in the forehead and works its way down the body, rarely reaching the toes. It is not dangerous. It is associated with the usual reddening of any flush as well as itching and irritation, but it does not cause sweating, as does the menopausal flush. No one should ever take niacin without being warned that this flush may occur. The first flush is the worst. After that, it gradually decreases in intensity until it is gone, unless the niacin is stopped for a day or two when the same sequence occurs. For many patients, the vasodilatation is a positive therapeutic effect.

Other possible side effects of vitamin B$_3$ are nausea, and if the dose is too high and the vitamin is not stopped, vomiting. In rare cases, it causes skin irritation. It does not cause liver damage, but it can elevate liver function tests. This does not mean there is underlying liver damage. The tests usually clear with continued use, and this elevation may be prevented by taking 1.2 grams of lecithin twice daily. Whether or not patients will tolerate the initial flush depends almost entirely on the physician. If the physician knows how to use niacin, the vast majority of patients will have little difficulty with it. The main side effects are positive, since it is one of the most important energy vitamins in the body.

Niacinamide does not normally cause flushing. However, in about 1 percent of the people who take it, there is a very unpleasant flush. If this occurs, the niacinamide must be stopped. Too high a dose will cause nausea and eventually vomiting.

The anticancer property of vitamin B_3 was discussed at a meeting in Texas in 1987 by Jacobson and Jacobson (1987), who studied the enzyme in the body that splits ADP (adenosine diphosphate) into ATP (adenosine triphosphate), the main chemical used for energy by cells. This enzyme is known as poly (ADP-ribose) polymerase, or poly (ADP) synthesase, or poly (ADP-ribose) transferase. It contains NAD (nicotinamide adenine dinucleotide), a form of vitamin B_3. When strands of DNA (deoxyribonucleic acid) are broken, the enzyme is activated, and it transfers NAD to the ADP-ribose polymer, where it helps repair the breaks and increases the cell's capacity to repair itself. Damage caused by any carcinogenic factor—such as radiation or chemicals—is thus to a degree neutralized or counteracted.

The NAD←—>NADH system is an essential component of the enzyme in the body that repairs broken, cut, or torn DNA molecules. DNA molecules can be torn by free radicals and by radiation. If they are not repaired rapidly, they tend to become cancerous.

Jacobson and Jacobson hypothesize that niacin prevents cancer. They treated two groups of human cells with carcinogens. The group given adequate niacin developed tumors at a rate only 10 percent of the rate in the group deficient in niacin. Dr. M. Jacobson is quoted as saying, "We know that diet is a major risk factor, that diet has both beneficial and detrimental components. What we cannot assess at this point is the optimal amount of niacin in the diet. The fact that we don't have pellagra does not mean we are getting enough niacin to confer resistance to cancer."

Vitamin B$_3$ may increase the therapeutic efficacy of anticancer treatments. In mice, niacinamide increased the toxicity of irradiation against tumors. It increased radiosensitivity in cancer of the head and neck from 10 to 80 percent by enhancing blood flow to the tumor. Nicotinamide also enhanced the effect of chemotherapy. Radiotherapy decreases the amount of NAD (nicotinamide adenine dinucleotide) in the liver by impairing the conversion of tryptophan to NAD. It would be prudent for every patient receiving radiation to take supplemental vitamin B$_3$. People exposed to irradiation from any source should add this supplement.

Vitamin B$_3$ has been shown to be involved in cancer. In animals, there is a direct relationship between the activity of nicotinamide methyl transferase (a form of vitamin B$_3$) in cells and the presence of cancer. In animals with cancer, there is increased destruction of nicotinamide, making less available to make enough of the NAD$\longleftrightarrow$NADH system. This finding applied to all tumors except the solid tumors, Lewis lung carcinoma, and melanoma B16.

In other cases, Gerson (1945,1949) treated a series of cancer patients with special diets and with some nutrients, including 50 mg of niacin eight to ten times per day. Dr. Gerson was the first physician to emphasize the use of multivitamins and some multiminerals.

Prof. James Kirkland, Department of Human Biology and Nutritional Science, University of Guelph, Canada, found in a series of excellent studies that niacin decreased the risk in rats of developing chemotherapy-induced leukemia and cancer of the bone marrow after treatment. Patients undergoing chemotherapy are 10 to 100 times more likely to develop these cancers, because they have too little NAD. NAD is the active anti-pellagra coenzyme. Kirkland suggests, "Pharmacological supplementation of niacin may represent a rapid and safe way to help protect the bone marrow cells of cancer patients." It is protective against DNA damage.

Additional evidence that vitamin B$_3$ is therapeutic for cancer arises from the National Coronary Study,

Canner (1986). Between 1966 and 1975, five drugs used to lower cholesterol levels were compared with a placebo in 8,341 men, ages thirty to sixty-four, who had suffered a myocardial infarction at least three months before entering the study. About 6,000 were alive at the end of the study. Nine years later, only niacin had decreased the death rate significantly from all causes. Mortality decreased 11 percent, and longevity increased by two years. The death rate from cancer was also decreased.

CHAPTER 6

VITAMIN E

Vitamin E includes the tocopherols, of which d-alpha tocopherol succinate has the most anti-cancer properties. It is the major lipid-soluble antioxidant, protecting the polyunsaturated fatty acids in membranes against peroxidation—the process by which fatty acids are oxidized through the action of an enzyme called peroxidase. The usual intake is about 12 IU (international units) daily. I have patients who take 800 IU daily. Vitamin E destroys nitrites, which have been shown to increase the incidence of cancer. It protects the red blood cells in lungs against the toxic effect of ozone, and from hydroxyl radical toxicity. K.N. Prasad (1999) reported that alpha tocopherol succinate induced differentiation in melanoma cells and inhibited the growth of neuroblastoma, rat glioma, and human prostate and melanoma cells.

> **Differentiation**
> *The process of changes by which cells become specialized in form and function. It is the degree to which a tumor resembles normal tissue. Well-differentiated tumors resemble normal tissue; the closer the resemblance, the better the prognosis.*

Recent studies have shown an inverse relationship between levels of vitamin E in blood and the development of cancer. Knekt, Aromaa, and Aaran (1991) examined alpha-tocopherol levels in 36,265 adults in Finland. After eight years, there were 766 cases of cancer. People with low levels of alpha tocopherol had one and a half times the chance of getting cancer compared with those with the highest level. This association was strongest with gastrointestinal cancers and other cancers not related to smoking. Other

---

Some Types of Cancers

Melanoma is a very aggressive cancer of the cells that produce pigment in the skin, that can spread to other areas of the body, including internal organs, if not detected and treated early.

Neuroblastoma is a malignant cancer that arises in immature nerve cells and affects mostly infants and children.

Glioma are the most common primary brain tumors, which begin in the supportive tissue of the brain. The most common gliomas are astrocytomas, ependymomas, oligodendrogliomas, and tumors with mixtures of two or more of these cell types.

Kaposi's sarcoma is a cancer that develops in connective tissue, causing tumors in the tissues below the skin surface or in the mucous membranes. It usually develops in association with illnesses such as human immunodeficiency virus (HIV) and acquired immunodeficiency syndrome (AIDS).

---

studies showed that lower vitamin E levels may be associated with lung cancer, and to a greater degree than the association of this disease with low levels of vitamin A.

The association between cancer and vitamin E consumption and cancer is not strong, but an increasing number of reports are showing that there is some connection. When so many variables are involved, it is very difficult to find very high correlations between the condition and the effect of only one nutrient. As long as we cannot be sure what the most effective cancer preventive agents and therapeutic compounds are, it seems only prudent to ensure that patients, as well as healthy individuals, are obtaining enough vitamin E.

CHAPTER 7

THE CAROTENOIDS
AND VITAMIN A

Most studies regarding the carotenoid beta-carotene and cancer found a relationship between the two. The Finnish Antioxidant and Lung Cancer Study appeared to show an increase in the incidence of lung cancer when low levels of beta-carotene were present. But interestingly, this is not what the dozens of authors of this study concluded. They found that beta-carotene did not decrease the incidence of lung cancer; on the contrary, there was a statistically insignificant increase among the beta-carotene group. It is, therefore, very important to know exactly the method used in this study.

The study used a large population of male smokers ages fifty to sixty-nine who were followed for five to eight years. One group was given the synthetic dl-alpha tocopherol. Another group was given 20 mg of beta-carotene, a third (control) group was on placebo, and the fourth group received both antioxidants. All the subjects had smoked five or more cigarettes daily for over thirty-five years. However, the beta-carotene group smoked one year more than the control group. How significant is one more year of heavy smoking for increasing the number of advanced lung cancers? The authors do not discuss this.

> **Placebo**
> An inactive substance or preparation used in controlled experiments testing the efficacy of another substance.

At the end of the study, men in the placebo group with the highest blood levels of these two antioxidants had the lowest incidence of lung cancer. In the dl-alpha tocopherol group, there was an insignificant 2 percent reduction in incidence of lung cancer (P =

0.8). In the beta-carotene group, there was an 18 percent increase in incidence. Out of 14,560 men on beta-carotene, 474 developed cancer, while 402 of 14,573 men not on beta-carotene developed cancer. The incidence of cancer increased from 2.76 percent for the control group to 3.26 percent for the treated group.

I suggest that this minor difference is not of clinical significance, even though it is statistically significant. However, in this statistically sophisticated study, dividing 3.26 by 2.76 yields the much larger number of 18 percent, which appears enormous. It will be the only figure the unwary reader will remember, and probably the only figure that will be used by the popular press. With large sample sizes such as these, a minor variation can easily become blown up to a major finding.

There must have been something very odd about that group of Finnish men. For one thing, the authors reported that 34 percent of the men on beta-carotene developed yellow skin. This is totally foreign to my experience. I have started at least 500 subjects on this amount of beta-carotene and more, and have never seen any yellowing of the skin with this dose, although I have seen some with higher doses. Does this mean that these heavy smokers had so compromised their livers that they could not deal with normal doses of beta-carotene? The authors do point out the many possible factors that might have given them these results, and the commentators also refer to them in an editorial in the same issue. These authors write, "Finally, study findings regarded as showing supplementation to be beneficial or harmful may occur by chance."

I consider this study to have proved nothing, except that if you give tiny doses of vitamin E to subjects nothing will happen, and if you give heavy chronic smokers 20 mg of beta-carotene their incidence of lung cancer will not change. Jack Challem reanalyzed the Finnish study, and concluded that alcohol, synthetic beta-carotene, and hasty conclusions may have created this study fiasco.

Cancer is probably present and undetectable in patients for a long time, perhaps many years, before it is finally discovered. The truly preventive study should therefore start long before any tumors have started, which could mean many years. With this large group of heavy smokers, it is certain that a significant fraction already had the cancer. This was, therefore, a mixed study consisting of: 1) treatment for those already with cancer; and 2) prevention for those who did not have any. Unfortunately, it will never be possible to say how much each group contributed. I would suggest that future studies start with a much younger population with much less chance of already having cancer.

The protective effect of dietary vitamin A against cancer was first reported in 1975. Since then, a large number of studies have consistently shown that higher levels of vitamin A in food are associated with decreased incidence of cancer. In vitro and animal studies have also found that vitamin A is protective against cancer. Vitamin A supplements have been used to potentiate the action of chemotherapy. There has been no outcry against using this antioxidant in combination with chemotherapy. In Japan, investigators used vitamin A, 5FU (Fluorouracil, a chemotherapy drug), and cobalt-60 radiation on hundreds of patients with head and neck tumors, which are particularly difficult to treat. The combination was very effective. In a study in Vancouver, Canada, 60 mg per week (nearly 200,000 IU) for six months led to complete remission in oral precancerous lesions in fifty-seven cases.

Potentiate
To increase the effect of, or action of, a drug or biochemical reaction.

Goodman concluded from a survey of the literature, ". . . that vitamin A and carotenoids are of considerable import to the prevention and treatment of many diverse cancers. In addition they are potentially valuable in potentiating and mitigating against many of the toxic effects of radiotherapy and chemotherapy."

CHAPTER 8

FOLIC ACID
(FOLATE)

Folic acid was one of the less interesting vitamins until Dr. Smithells in Scotland showed that giving pregnant women folic acid at the beginning of their pregnancy substantially decreased the incidence of neural tube defects (NTD). The possibility that folic acid was involved in these defects was first suggested in 1964. Dr. R.W. Smithells showed that giving pregnant women extra folic acid decreased the incidence of NTDs in 1989. Before that, he had measured the red blood cell folate and white blood cell vitamin C levels of mothers who had babies with NTDs, and found that they were low in both nutrients. It was thus known since 1989 that a multivitamin preparation containing folic acid would decrease the number of babies with neural tube defects. This finding should have been greeted with enthusiasm, but it was not.

The objection to Smithells' work arose from the pervasive belief that folic acid was dangerous if patients had pernicious anemia. This is why higher dose folic acid pills must be given as prescriptions. Hunter wrote:

> Indeed, it became part of medical dogma that folate could precipitate more severe and aggressive neurologic complications. Dickinson did a comparison of case studies and series of patients with B_{12} deficiency, before and after the introduction of treatment with folic acid, and found no evidence that folate increased the rate or the severity of the neurologic presentation of B_{12} deficiency. About 28 per cent of cases of B_{12} deficiency present neurologically, and practicing physicians

should always consider this diagnosis in a patient with paresthesia, weakness, or ataxia. Dickinson considered it absurd to withhold supplements because some patients with pernicious anemia might not be sick enough to be diagnosed by their physician. Because there is a very remote risk I also have my patient take a vitamin B-complex 50's preparation which provides 50 micrograms of this vitamin daily.

In the United States, 25,000 babies were born each year with these congenital defects. The number is probably much lower now, with the addition of folic acid to flour. It has been estimated that each child in Canada with this condition costs about $40,000 in medical and surgical care by the time he or she is twelve years old. I assume costs would be the same in the United States. Taking very small amounts of folic acid decreases the incidence of NTD by about 75 percent. This means that if these women had known about the value of this vitamin and had taken it, there would have been only 6,000 babies born with NTDs—that's a saving of about one-quarter of a billion dollars each year in health care. The cost of the folic acid is pennies per day. But due to the skepticism and resistance of the profession, which would not act until several double-blind trials had been completed, these facts were not made known, and for too many years, the disease was allowed to run rampant. This twenty-year delay cost the United States healthcare system $5 billion. That is the cost of delay, or skepticism, when there was no scientific reason to be afraid of this gentle and safe vitamin. Even if the folic acid had not been proven to prevent neural tube defects, there was no danger from taking 1 mg of this vitamin daily until the final convincing evidence was obtained.

Treatments that decrease folic acid levels increase the risk of developing neural tube defect. This includes anticonvulsants and the atypical antipsychotics. Schizophrenic women who take these antipsychotics have a higher risk of having babies with neural tube defects.

Folic acid has antitumor properties. This includes prevention of stomach, colorectal, and cervical cancers, according to Rampersaud, Bailey, and Kauwell (2002). A study in Western Australia found mothers who used folate supplements and iron had more than a 60 percent reduction in risk of having children develop acute lymphoblastic leukemia. The risk was reduced only 25 percent with iron supplements alone. According to recent Canadian studies, there is also a 50 percent decrease in the risk of giving birth to children who develop neuroblastoma with folate supplementation. An unexpected benefit of adding folic acid to flour is the decrease incidence of neuroblastoma from one in 6,000 births to one in 12,000 births. Higher doses than those obtained from flour probably would decrease the incidence of this cancer even more. Authors following the vitamin-as-prevention paradigm do not recommend using high-dose supplemental folic acid. It takes a lot of clinical evidence before they are willing to jump into the vitamins-as-treatment paradigm. However, folate has been used safely in 25 to 50 mg doses for treating depression. It makes sense that if a nutrient can prevent something, and if it is safe when used in higher doses than can be found in foods, that it might also have some treatment value.

CHAPTER 9

VITAMIN D

Without enough vitamin D_3 (the biologically active form of vitamin D), we get rickets. But rickets should have disappeared long ago. We know that this vitamin is made in the skin on exposure to ultraviolet light, and that it is readily available in fish liver oils, particularly in halibut liver oil and in smaller concentrations in cod liver oil. Cod liver oil given to children, in spite of its bad taste, was a special spring event for many families. This seems to have vanished as a spring habit, but many of my patients still remember how their mothers forced them to take the foul-tasting substance.

Rickets
A nutritional disease caused by not getting enough vitamin D. This interferes with the ability of the body to absorb calcium and causes softening and deformation of the bones.

Rickets was caused by ignorance then, and it's coming back again, due to ignorance of a different kind. This time, it is an iatrogenic disease caused by advice from the medical profession, especially by dermatologists. They have become extremely fearful of ultraviolet radiation as a cause of skin cancer, specifically the melanomas. This fear, and their advice to stay out of the sun, to use sun screens, and to keep their children covered at all times has had the unintended consequence that rickets is once more becoming a public health problem. Canadian doctors are seeing more cases of childhood rickets, and apparently this num-

Iatrogenic
A medical problem, adverse condition, or unfavorable response induced inadvertently by the medical or surgical treatment of a physician.

ber is increasing each year. In the past two years, there have been eighty-four reported cases of rickets in Canada. Three generations ago this disease was so rare that rickets was considered a medical curiosity. Once considered an old disease of the nineteenth century, when children were malnourished or forced to work in dark mines and factories, rickets is again being seen in Great Britain, the United States, Australia, and Canada. Canadian pediatricians are recommending that vitamin D supplements be used in addition to what is present in breast milk and in other foods. Perhaps the pediatricians should talk more to the dermatologists.

The Cancer Council of New South Wales in Australia rejects the explanation that this problem is due to lack of sun. They maintain that ten minutes exposure to sun three times each week is enough to maintain healthy vitamin D levels. But how do they explain the resurgence of rickets? Perhaps if they jumped out of the old vitamin-as-prevention paradigm and into the new paradigm, they would understand that blood levels may not correlate well with clinical findings. There are simple precautionary measures with respect to exposure to sun without denying children the benefits of sun and of vitamin D (see Burke, Combs and Gross in the section under selenium). I recommend the following vitamin cocktail to prevent sunburn and melanoma: 200 micrograms of selenium daily, 800 IU daily of vitamin E, the body's best fat-soluble antioxidant, and 1 to 3 grams daily of vitamin C, the best water-soluble antioxidant, in addition to reasonable precautions against excess sun tanning such as not lying on the beach in California for ten hours daily.

Resurgence of rickets is not the only problem that occurs with a lack of vitamin D. Vitamin D has anticancer properties as well. Evidence has been available for the past fifty years that regular sun exposure is associated with decreases in death rates from cancer. Dark-skinned people who move to areas lacking sun are more frequently hit by cancer. In areas of the United States that are exposed to less ultraviolet, rates increase for prostate, breast, and colon cancer. H.D. Foster (1992) suggests this involves calcium metabolism. Twice as many women with breast cancer have a variant vitamin D gene, and variant genes require higher doses of vitamin. This suggests that vitamin D ought to be used in the treatment of some forms of cancer, especially prostate, breast, and colon cancer.

This conclusion is supported by the results of further analysis from the recent Cancer Prevention Study II Nutrition Cohort involving 127,749 adults. Calcium supplementation and vitamin D intake offered some protection from colon cancer. This case control study compared nutrient intake in 1992 in the 683 subjects who developed colon cancer during the following five years with intake in those who did not develop it. Calcium intake from supplements was inversely related to colon cancer incidence. There was no significant association with dairy product intake.

The usual small doses of vitamin D that most people take are not adequate. One day in the sun in California will synthesize 10,000 units in the skin. I recommend 2,000 to 4,000 IU daily, using both one of the fish oils and the pure vitamin D tablets. Embry recommends 4,000 to 6,000 IU as the optimal daily intake.

CHAPTER 10

ESSENTIAL
FATTY ACIDS

The connection between essential fatty acids and cancer has been described in a huge number of published studies. One of the leaders in this field, Dr. David Horrobin, was also a leader in having evening primrose oil, and later fish oils, examined clinically both for prevention and treatment of cancer. I did not add essential oils to my program for many years except for flaxseed oil, following the work of Dr. Johanna Budwig, in Europe, who considered it a major part of her treatment for cancer.

Essential Fatty Acids and Cancer

The relationship between essential fatty acids and cancer is not clear because there are so many essential fatty acids. The two main series are the omega-6 and omega-3 series. While some of these fatty acids appear to be beneficial, some may not be. The saturated fats, which have suffered a bad reputation, are coming back in for consideration and may also play a major role. Studies on prevention in animals or in vitro studies suggest that the essential fatty acids do play a role in cancer. In one double-blind clinical study, ten patients with sporadic colorectal polyps were given fish oil. The results indicated that fish oil could protect against the development of colon cancer. And fish oil could also help deal with cachexia—the severe terminal weight loss in some cancer patients. At the Edinburgh Royal Infirmary, two groups of pancreatic cancers were studied. The one group was given a high-calorie/high-protein diet, and the second group a high-calorie/high-protein liquid diet supplemented with omega-3 essential fatty acids and vitamins E and C. Before the study, these patients were losing an average of 6.6 pounds each month. All of the patients stopped losing weight, but the patients who consumed most of their drink gained the most, and these patients were only in the group receiving the supplements. Not all the credit can be given to the essential fatty acids, however, since the patients were also given vitamin E and vitamin C.

The use of the essential fatty acids will do no harm and may be very helpful. Given the present information, I think that one should consider using ground flaxseed, fresh flaxseed oil with lots of vitamin E, or the fish oils to deal with free-radical formation. Also, one need not avoid saturated fats. These are turning out to be not as bad as many previously thought they were. However, trans-fatty acids, also called "trans fats," should be rigorously avoided. They are present in hydrogenated fats/oils and in much of the processed foods available today.

CHAPTER 11

SELENIUM

It is difficult to establish strong correlations between any diseases and any one nutrient when a large number of nutrient factors are involved. H.D. Foster (1992) in his excellent review concluded that the evidence for a negative correlation between selenium intake and the incidence of cancer was strong. In one twenty-seven-country survey, breast cancer mortality correlated strongly and negatively with dietary selenium. However, case control studies yield conflicting data. Some workers find no difference in blood selenium levels between breast cancer cases and controls, while others find they are low in the cancer cases. Prospective studies also yield mixed data. One study on 4,480 subjects, of whom 111 developed cancer, showed a significant but small decrease in selenium in the patients who developed cancer.

More recent reviews confirmed Foster's conclusion. A study by Cornell University and University of Arizona showed that patients taking selenium had a 41 percent less chance of getting cancer compared with those taking a placebo. The treated group experienced 18 percent less mortality. Wahrendorf, Munoz, and Lu (1988) supplemented the diet of people living in a high-risk area in China for esophageal cancer. They found that at the end of the trial, individuals who showed large increases in retinol, riboflavin, and zinc blood levels were more likely to have normal esophagus tissues when they were microscopically studied. Yu, Mao, Xiao, et al. (1990) gave 300 micrograms of selenium to forty healthy miners in a double-blind experiment to test its safety. They concluded that this use of selenium was safe and effective in humans with low selenium status, and that selenium protected lymphocytes against DNA damage. *Cancer Research* announced on June 15, 2003, that some genes were related to incidence of breast cancer and that these genes were less responsive to selenium stimulation. Over a hundred animal and dozens of epidemiological studies linked high selenium state with decreased risk of cancer. On February 21, 2003, the Food and Drug Administration announced the validity of two health claims: (1) selenium may reduce the risk of certain cancers, and (2) selenium may produce anti-carcinogenic effects in the body.

Lymphocytes
Type of small white blood cell found in blood, lymph nodes, spleen, and bone marrow that fight infection and disease.

Selenium and Skin Cancer

As mentioned previously, the frequent and recurring reports in the news media about the dangers inherent in excessive exposure to sunlight continually remind and frighten some people about the possibility of getting skin cancer. However, these reports do not discuss the connection between the nutritional health of the population and their susceptibility to cancer of the skin. Since ultraviolet radiation increases the formation of free radicals, it would not be surprising that increasing the intake of antioxidants could prevent some of the toxic reactions to ultraviolet radiation. Selenium is an example of such a preventive nutrient.

Burke, Combs, Gross, (1992) reported that selenium given to hairless pigmented mice protected them against damage from ultraviolet irradiation. They found that both a lotion containing 0.02% of L-selenomethionine and an oral administration of water containing 1.2 ppm (parts per million) of selenium were protective. These dosages did not cause any toxic reactions. They concluded that, "SeMet is effective in protecting against skin cancer induced by UV irradiation, both by retarding the onset and reducing the number of lesions." These formulas were also ". . . effective in reducing the acute damage induced by UV irradiation-inflammation (sun-burn), blistering, and pigmentation (tanning)." No blisters developed in the treated mice during early weeks of irradiation, but they did develop in two-thirds of the control mice. The report concluded with the practical suggestion that ". . . protection might be provided by either topically or orally administered SeMet." In a subsequent report, Burke (1992) con-firmed these findings. She reported that both oral and topical selenium supplementation decreased the incidence and chronic damage from ultraviolet irradiation without being toxic. Mice treated with selenium had a delayed onset and a markedly lesser incidence of skin cancer.

Selenium is a good antioxidant. It is synergistic with vitamin E, the body's best-known fat-soluble antioxidant. The daily recommended dose is 200 micrograms. I have given 600 micrograms and more to certain patients for many years, and have seen no toxic side effects. I would, therefore, suggest that the three best-known natural antioxidants, vitamin C, vitamin E, and selenium, be used to protect people against the toxic effect of excessive ultraviolet irradi-ation. The dose would be 200 micrograms of selen-ium, 800 IU of vitamin E, and 3 or more grams of vitamin C per day. It should not take too much time to test these antioxidants in controlled studies, but because the danger from ultraviolet-induced skin cancer and melanoma is potentially so great, it would be prudent to take these simple nutrients as a pre-caution. They would, of course, have other advan-tages as well.

Selenium and HIV/AIDS

Selenium also plays a much more important role in the virus diseases that plague the world today. HIV/AIDS is the worst, and SARS is another that has appeared in the news even more recently. People who have HIV and AIDS are much more susceptible to some cancers, particularly Kaposi's sarcoma, so pre-venting AIDS will also decrease the incidence of can-cer. Foster (2002) summarized the evidence that the real cause of AIDS is a deficiency of selenium, more accurately, a deficiency of glutathione peroxidase. The evidence is very powerful. Glutathione peroxidase is one of the very important antioxidant enzymes in the body. Any HIV virus introduced into the body quickly binds to this enzyme, and if a person is short of selenium, this binding causes a selenium deficiency. This deficiency is responsible for the multiple symptoms and signs of AIDS by compromising the immune system and making the individual more susceptible to a host of other diseases, including cancer and tuberculosis. If the person has enough selenium, the HIV virus will do little damage and the virus and the individual can coexist.

A remarkable example of this is Senegal, a small country in Africa. In Senegal, there are no precautions against infection. The capital is rife with prostitutes, and it is a favorite attraction for men from all parts of Africa. The men do not use condoms. In Senegal, the incidence of HIV is about 1 percent of the population, the same today as it was about twenty years ago. The countries around Senegal had an incidence as high as 40 percent, although this has more recently stabilized around 15 to 20 percent. According to Foster, the reason for the difference in HIV rates is that Senegal's soil is very rich in selenium, while the soil in the other countries is not. Therefore, if you take in enough selenium, you are not as apt to become infected with HIV, and if you are infected, it is less likely to progress to AIDS. Foster suggested that giving these four nutrients—selenium, cysteine, glutamine, and tryptophan—would be therapeutic for AIDS, and in a few cases, he described its therapeutic value. This is very exciting work. AIDS thus appears to be a multiple dependency since all four nutrients are needed. The easiest to supplement is selenium, which can be put in the water, as is done in China in some regions, and into food as has been done for the past fifty years in the United States and Canada with niacinamide, riboflavin, and thiamine. The selenium requirement is 200 micrograms daily.

CHAPTER 12

ZINC AND COPPER

Zinc deficiency induces immunosuppression. Thymus-dependent acquired immunity—that is, immunity that is not provided automatically by the body, but develops by being exposed to a particular disease—is most severely affected. Zinc plays a large number of roles in the defense responses of the body. These are: 1) it contributes to plasma's ability to resist attack, 2) it is important to the cell's ability to bind to and utilize enzymes and nutrients, 3) in high concentration, it inhibits the function of phagocytes, small white blood cells that fight infections and protect the body from diseases it has been exposed to, 4) low body stores of zinc are associated with dysfunction of T cells, 5) the synthesis of nucleic acid and protein, two critical substances for the body, is dependent on zinc, and 6) zinc plays a key role in metalloenzyme function (enzymes that contain a metal ion). These roles may explain some of the anticarcinogenic effects of zinc.

Phagocytes
Cells that engulf and destroy particles such as bacteria, protozoa, and other organisms, aged red blood cells, and cellular debris.

When the body is zinc deficient, the spleen and thymus decrease in weight, lymphocyte count is reduced, the body's response to antigens (foreign substances) is decreased, immunoglobulin levels are decreased, T-cell helper function is interfered with, and susceptibility to infection is increased. It should

Immunoglobulin
Proteins in the body that bind to invading organisms and destroy them, acting as antibodies to fight infection.

not be surprising that zinc deficiency is related to cancer, and that treatment with zinc may be therapeutic.

Foster (1992) examined the correlation between breast cancer and several soil constituents. For the years 1950 to 1967 in the United States, there was a negative correlation between cancer incidence and very low zinc levels in soils, meaning that the incidence of breast cancer was higher where there was less zinc supplied in the soil and therefore in the local food supply.

There is an inverse relationship between copper and zinc. A deficiency in the body of one of these elements will cause an increase in the amount of the other. The easiest way to bring down copper levels is to increase the intake of zinc. Fortunately, zinc is a very safe trace mineral and can be given in useful dosages for long periods of time with hardly any side effects.

With all this evidence of the importance of zinc, I decided to include adequate zinc in the supplemental program for the cancer patients who came to me for nutritional advice. I used the following compounds and daily dosages for these patients: zinc sulfate 220 mg, zinc gluconate 50 mg, or zinc citrate 50 mg.

CHAPTER 13

THE THERAPEUTIC
PROGRAM

We can no longer ignore the extensive data that is already available in the medical literature regarding the orthomolecular therapy and the value of vitamins in cancer treatment. This data contains conclusions of independent physicians with no ties to the drug industry. They have not sought fame and fortune by their studies, and their only goal was to improve the results of treatment for their patients. They did not have the support of the medical research establishment, or the large grants needed by institutions before they perform clinical studies. They didn't do prospective randomized controlled experiments because they didn't have the resources, financial or otherwise. But their clinical data is every bit as strong, perhaps much stronger, than the data accepted by the medical community from the early noncontrolled studies on the modern tranquilizers when they first came into use between 1950 and 1960. By the end of 1960, we knew that these powerful drugs were active. The controlled experiments that followed simply confirmed what was already general knowledge. Why were these uncontrolled studies accepted while the studies on vitamins are ignored? The difference is that the drug companies poured millions into promoting their patented tranquilizer compounds, and no one is doing the same for orthomolecular treatment of cancer, because vitamins can't be patented.

My conclusions are based upon observations of nearly 1,300 patients that I have treated since 1977, as well as on the published studies. My conclusions are plausible, perhaps stronger than that, and approaching a level of certainty indicating that it will be doing patients a disservice to withhold this form of treatment while we wait for the conclusive large-scale studies that will be conducted over the next ten years. I have recommended it to members of my family and to friends. I hope that you will come to the same conclusion after you have read and studied the information presented in this book, and have read some of the books and papers dealing with cancer. If enough interested patients and their loved ones become educated and demand these treatment options, it will stimulate the large-scale studies needed to provide the type of proof a skeptical medical establishment demands. We cannot wait too long. Remember the enormous cost of waiting that happened before pregnant women were given folic acid to prevent neural tube abnormalities.

The Patients

Family doctors, general practitioners, surgeons, or other specialists refer all of my patients to me. I do not see walk-ins. Because I am a psychiatrist, doctors would not refer nonpsychiatric patients to me. This meant that physically ill patients had great difficulty persuading their doctors to make that referral. When they were referred, it meant that the referring physician concluded that I could be helpful, both because I am a psychiatrist and because I was practicing orthomolecular psychiatry. It is easy to understand that most patients diagnosed with cancer will suffer from anxiety, depression, or usually both, especially if they are told it is terminal or if they have been declared treatment failures.

I had nothing to do with the patients' original diagnoses or their standard treatment. In most cases, they had already completed their standard treatment, or were in the process of completing it, or had failed to respond and no longer qualified for additional treatment. When they were advised by the cancer clinic that they were no longer treatable, they became depressed and anxious, and sought referral to me. They still remained under the care of their family doctor. At the beginning of my experience with cancer patients, most were self-referred, meaning that it was the patients' idea that they see me and they asked their doctors to make the referral. Some of them were very forceful and demanding, and a few patients changed their doctors in order to obtain a referral. One patient at the end of her interview with her doctor after her treatment asked whether she could get another appointment. He replied, "There is no point. You will be dead in one week." She became depressed and her husband, who was with her, became very angry. They demanded that the doctor immediately refer her to me, which he did. She lived another thirty months.

If patients asked whether they should depend only on the use of vitamins, I replied that I had no experience using the orthomolecular approach without the concurrent use of standard treatment, and that I could not advise them. Only a handful of patients refused standard treatment. There were some who desperately needed surgery, radiation, or chemotherapy and who refused to accept this until I advised them that in my opinion it was essential. Many had been told that the orthomolecular treatment would interfere with their standard treatment, and several specialists told patients that if they insisted on using vitamins they would no longer treat them. (The issue of the impact of antioxidant therapy on chemotherapy and radiation was discussed earlier.)

Each patient was seen at least twice. The first visit was used to determine whether their depression or anxiety required psychiatric treatment. The second visit, usually two months later, was used to make sure the program was followed and to answer questions. I did not see most of the patients after that. I think that I should have followed them up more often, however, and I believe the results would have been even better if I had done so.

The Whole Treatment Program

When treating schizophrenic patients, the treatment must include adequate shelter (not the streets), good nutrition, the patient-doctor relationship (respect and support), and medical orthomolecular treatment. Using the first three modalities alone will help 50 percent of these patients recover. The same four modalities are essential in the treatment of cancer or any illness.

The Importance of the Patient-Doctor Relationship

The relationship between patient and doctor is fundamental to the treatment process for all illnesses. Patients must trust that the doctor will do everything possible to help him or her gain relief from discomforts. As with any enduring relationship, the trust is reinforced by the interaction. This is true for all medical and psychiatric illnesses, and even more so when the disease is life threatening like cancer.

My rule is that patients should leave their doctor's office feeling better, not worse. Too often have I been told that they went to their oncologist for the interview full of hope that they would find a solution with the oncologist's help. They left feeling totally defeated by the information they were given, the way it was presented to them, and the attitude of the doctor. The doctor must have the knowledge the patient needs, the interest in helping them, and should be able to impart a level of hope, for without hope, patients will get worse. My criticism of many oncologists and cancer radiation specialists is that patients leave their offices feeling worse, not better. I do not imply that the doctor has to be dishonest if there is little chance for recovery. It is necessary to leave hope even when the prognosis is very grim, however, for without hope the patient's full defenses against the disease cannot be mobilized. For example, the patient has a serious illness such as lung cancer, for which there may be a 5 percent probability of surviving two years. The usual oncologist will tell the patient that the chance of dying is 95 percent. If the doctor presents it another way, and advises his patient that he has a 5 percent chance of surviving, he allows the patient to have some hope. I reinforce this by telling my patients case histories of patients who against all the odds have survived. Patients are intelligent. They know the prognosis is not good, but they also know there is a chance. People want and will believe in that chance, which is why so many buy lottery tickets, where the chance of winning a million is much less than the chance of surviving the major cancers. I discuss my patients' survival evidence from my orthomolecular practice. I encourage my patients to take a very active role in their treatment, and when they come up with ideas that I know are not harmful, I encourage them to go ahead. I want my patients to become very involved in their treatment and become the active manager. My role is to advise, and not to give orders. We are equals, except the patient is suffering personally, and I suffer with them.

Usually, there is a collegial relationship between the family doctors and the specialist to whom they have been referring their patients. The specialist recommends an approach, and the family doctor supports that approach. The patient is not confronted with conflicting advice from two doctors. But because orthomolecular medicine is still so unique, many referring doctors who made the referral under great pressure did not provide the support their patients needed. As previously mentioned, some would try to persuade their patients not to take any vitamins. Many patients would then change doctors. Many doctors refused to refer their patients to me, and some told their patients that I was not practicing anymore, that I was dead, that I would charge too much, that I would order them not to use medication, and more. In fact, I do not think I am dead, I am still practicing, I work within the provincial plan so Canadian patients do not have to pay anything to see me, and I look upon orthomolecular treatment as complementary to standard treatment. Sadly, patients find themselves caught in the middle, and don't receive the support they would get from their family doctors if they had not started on an orthomolecular treatment program.

The Cancer Clinic

The Cancer Clinic provides free cancer treatment to all British Columbia residents. I have free access to their charts on all of the patients I have seen. At first, the clinic was very suspicious of my motives and refused to let me see the charts unless I agreed that they could censor any reports or papers that I published. When I refused to allow this, they withdrew their objection, and I was able to see any charts I needed with the patient's permission. They routinely sent me follow-up reports, which entered my own files and were available to judge progress. A few oncologists referred their patients to me.

Quality of Life

The orthomolecular program enhances the quality of life. This is not surprising, since the use of vitamins improves the quality of life of almost every patient. Being sick is very stressful, and stress increases the utilization and loss of vitamins, especially the water-soluble ones. A professor of oncology who began to add vitamin C to his program was impressed with how quickly his patients responded. Before that, they all were sallow, haggard, as is typical with chemotherapy patients. This changed in one day when the vitamin was added, and they appeared much healthier and felt better. Many of my patients' families came to thank me after their spouse or parent died, because there was such a marked improvement in quality of life until they died. This was very comforting to their relatives.

Follow-Up Procedures

Patients were followed by calling the patients or their families, by contacting the referring doctors and/or the Cancer Clinic, and by following the obituaries in the local newspaper. Most of my patients came from Vancouver Island, and the local paper is the main paper in which these obituaries appeared. I followed each patient for at least ten years. If they had a recurrence of cancer, they would come back to see me

again. If they continued to suffer from a mood disor-
der, they would continue to see me until they were
well. A few patients had been under my care before
their cancer was diagnosed and they continued with
their previous treatment.

Overall Survival Rates of Patients Following the Program

I used survival as my criterion for response, because
it is hard data with which no one can argue. Tracking
started the day the patient first saw me after he
or she had been diagnosed as having cancer, and
stopped the day the person died, but I could not
determine the cause of death. Not all of the deaths
were due to their cancer.

The first series, reported with Linus Pauling, included 134 patients. Of this group, 101 were treated
using the orthomolecular program, and the others
were on standard treatment. From the group on orthomolecular treatment, 40 percent were alive ten years
later. Not one survived from the group on standard
treatment. From all patients seen between 1978 and
1993, 518 were on treatment; of this group, 40 percent survived five years and remained alive until the
end of ten years. From the standard treatment group,
6 percent survived ten years.

The following table shows the follow-up results of
my treated group and the control group (standard
treatment only).

	Treated (N 992)			Control (N 165)		
Years Alive	1	2	5	1	2	5
Number Alive	634	431	208	21	11	6

N = number of patients

CHAPTER 14

CLINICAL RESULTS OF ORTHOMOLECULAR TREATMENT

In this chapter, I will describe the outcome of treatment of a few of the more important types of cancer and a few case histories from each group to illustrate the outcome of treatment. We have to take into account that the patients who came to see me were self-selected and very highly motivated when we consider the results of the treatment. They had to be motivated, to escape from the box of only standard treatment from practitioners who are members of the chemotherapy and radiation faith. It took exceptional courage and determination to face their doctors and their oncologists and arrange to be referred.

Most of the patients were terminal, or they had been informed that there was nothing more that could be done and that there was no hope except for palliative treatment. This removal of hope prompted the break from classical medicine. These results experienced by these patients cannot be compared with the whole universe of cancer patients with similar types of tumors. They can be compared to my patients who could not follow my program for at least two months. I had concluded that a fair test of the program would demand at least two months of treatment, in the same way that one chemotherapy session would not be considered a fair test of chemotherapy if eight treatments were required. The patients who did break out of the box of traditional medicine's prognosis for them were rewarded by a positive attitude, by support,

Palliative
To relieve symptoms or offer comfort (such as relieving pain) without fixing or curing the underlying disease.

by attention to diet, by the use of nutrients, and by an improved quality of life.

My control group represents the level of illness of the entire group of my patients, who were all on standard treatment and had not responded. They remained under good standard care even after they came to see me.

I have not included the case histories of patients who did not respond to treatment. My patients suffered from the negative attitudes of their oncologist and radiologists, and I don't want to add the same burden to the readers of this book. I describe only positive responders, in the same way that I use these case histories to encourage my patients. I don't exaggerate response rates, and I provide the actual percentage of my patients from each group who lived five years. My patients are already well aware of their prognosis by the time they get to my office. I follow the rule that patients should leave me feeling better, not worse.

Under each type, I give the survival data and one or two case histories of recoveries to illustrate what has occurred.

Cancer of the Lung

The number of patients surviving by years is shown below.

Survival Rate	1 Year	2 Years	5 Years
Orthomolecular Treatment—N 63	23	11	5
Standard Treatment—N 18	0	0	0

Case History: Patient #37

Patient #37 was born in 1927. She was first seen in May 1981 and was alive more than ten years after diagnosis and referral to me.

Patient #37 felt sharp right-sided chest pain December 1980. X ray showed a large mass in her right lung. Bronchoscopic examination showed a visible tumor involving the lateral wall of the right lower lobe bronchus, extending into the right upper bronchus and occluding the orifice of the superior segment of her right lower lung. Biopsies were consistent with small cell (oat cell) bronchiogenic carcinoma. There were no metastases, but there was an ill-defined area of uptake in the left temporal-parietal region of the brain. Surgery was contraindicated.

Radiation therapy to the metastatic lesion in the brain was started in January 1981, followed by four courses of chemotherapy that were completed in June 1981. This was followed by a course of radiotherapy to the primary tumor site. This was competed in July 1981. The Cancer Clinic noted, "She understands it's palliative and not curative."

I recommended she take the following:

- Ascorbic acid: 4 grams three times daily
- Niacinamide: 500 mg three times daily
- A multivitamin preparation once daily

She followed her program for several months. When she was interviewed in August 1989, she could not remember having seen me. She was on the program for a few months only, and she continued to smoke. Her family doctor reported that she had always had a memory problem and that it had gotten worse following irradiation to her brain. At autopsy, the old lesions was healed, but a new site had developed a couple of months earlier and was rampant.

Cancer of the Colon

The number of patients surviving by years is shown below.

Survival Rate	1 Year	2 Years	5 Years
Orthomolecular Treatment—N 51	33	27	7
Standard Treatment—N 14	2	0	0

Cancer of the Breast

The number of patients surviving by years is shown as follows.

Survival Rate	1 Year	2 Years	
Orthomolecular Treatment—N 154	134	89	53 (5 years)
Standard Treatment—N 14	4	1	1 (3 years)

Sarcomas

Sarcomas appear to be more responsive to treatment. The first patient I saw in 1960 had Ewing's sarcoma of the arm, and was on the waiting list for surgery to amputate her arm. Her mother was a patient of mine being treated for depression, and she arranged for me to see her daughter. I started her on 1 gram of vitamin C three times daily and 1 gram of niacin three times daily. After one month, the surgery was canceled, and she remained well thereafter.

Ewing's Sarcoma
A cancer that starts in the bone or soft tissues. It is most common between the ages of ten and twenty. It appears most often on the pelvis, the thigh, and the trunk of the body.

The following table shows the results of treatment of twelve consecutive sarcoma patients who were seen beginning in 1980 and ending in 1999. Five died, living on the average 3.5 years. Seven are alive, average 7.8 years.

Patient Number	Year Born	Sex	Year of Onset	1st Year Seen	Present Condition	Years Alive
6	1908	M	1978	1980	Died 8/1989	9
22	1965	F	1979	1981	Alive	22
495	1957	M	1991	1993	Died 6/1998	5
647	1957	M	1994	1995	Alive	8
890	1929	F	1997	1997	Alive	6
916	1951	M	1997	1997	Alive	6
1019	1935	M	1998	1998	Died 4/2000	2
1027	1969	F	1998	1999	Alive	4

Patient Number	Year Born	Sex	Year of Onset	1st Year Seen	Present Condition	Years Alive
1035	1931	M	1998	1999	Died 9/2000	1
1039	1958	M	1998	1999	Alive	4
1040	1952	M	1998	1999	Alive	4
1091	1967	M	1998	1999	Died 11/2000	1

Case History: Patient #6

Patient #6, age seventy-two, was first seen in January 1980, and died of heart disease in July 1989. He had a triple bypass a few years before his death.

A stabbing pain in the left groin started in March 1978. A slow growing neurofibrosarcoma of the left groin was discovered and partially removed the following February. A course of palliative cobalt irradiation was applied to the left hip area during March 1979. The Cancer Clinic noted that "There is apparently residual tumor about the size of a grapefruit involving the left side of the pelvis and it was felt that it might be possible to give this man a course of cobalt irradiation on the off chance that this lesion might be radiosensitive although we do not expect this histologically to be particularly radiosensitive." There was some improvement in the swelling of the left leg and left groin following the radiotherapy, but a persistent infection developed at the operative site, which was treated with antibiotics. The Clinic noted in January 1980 that there had been some increased extension (enlargement) in the lower part of the left groin.

Patient #6 was very depressed, not only because of his cancer, but because his wife had terminal cancer and had just gone to the hospital. He had been looking after her by himself for the previous three months. He told his family doctor that he had a little money saved and that he would go to Mexico and blow it all if necessary. His family doctor then referred him to me. His wife died.

I advised him to start on the living diet, fruits, vegetables, and a minimum of meat. His supplements included:

- Vitamin C: 4 grams three times daily
- Niacinamide: 500 mg three times daily
- Pyridoxine: 250 mg three times daily
- Zinc gluconate: 100 mg daily
- A multimineral preparation

He could not increase his oral vitamin C dose because he developed loose stools. His physician gave him sodium ascorbate 2.5 grams intravenously three times a week starting in February 1980 until September 1980. A radiology report stated, "Comparison is made with the previous study of February 1979, which showed an apparent expanding destructive lesion involving the superior ramous of the left pubic bone which was involved with Paget's disease compatible with sarcomata's cancer of Paget's. Present study shows marked improvement with some apparent bony reconstruction of the left superior pubic ramus. There has certainly been no further bony destruction in the interior." The patient remained vigorously active until his death nine years later.

On May 5, 1980, he wrote: "Through out the period of treatment I have felt exceptionally fit and vital. The enclosed copy of a recent X ray is, to say the least, very encouraging. I have recently bought a new house, am going on a trip to Europe and am looking forward to a new happy healthful life." He remarried in 1981.

Case History: Patient #1039

Patient #1039 was born in 1958 and first seen on March 10, 1999. In 1984, while training in Victoria, he developed pain in the left pubic area. This was later diagnosed as a stress fracture, and subsequently a cyst was found. He would often have a sensation of tightness in his left groin after that, and he would have to stretch prior to activities.

For the following year and a half, he had increasing left groin pain, which sometimes wakened him at night. Occasionally, he would have pain shooting down the front of the leg to his ankle. He also noticed some weakness in his hip. He was still training eight to twelve hours per week because he had been competing in triathlons, and also had been coaching cyclists in Japan and Canada.

An X ray of the pelvis revealed a large bony mass 10 by 15 centimeters, arising from the left inferior and superior pubic rami. The tumor had not spread. He was waiting further examination with a biopsy to determine exactly what kind of a growth he had.

The radiologist reported a large exophytic mass arising posteriorly from the left side of the pubis, approximately 8 by 5 centimeters, displacing the bladder and rectum to the right. Extensive lytic changes were seen in the posterior aspect of the mass breaking through the cortex. It looked like a large osteochondroma with malignant degeneration. The cancer agency stated it was most likely he would require a resection of the lesion, which might include an internal left hemipelvectomy and a hip arthrodesis.

Following this diagnosis, he was advised to have surgery immediately, and a bed was booked for him. He refused, since losing half his pelvis would destroy his career and leave him with a quality of life he did not want to endure. He flew to Toronto to see another surgeon, who promptly gave him the same advice. He rejected that too, and came back to Victoria to start an orthomolecular program.

I advised him to follow the following program:

- Ascorbic acid: 4 grams taken four times daily, to be increased to sublaxative levels

- Niacinamide: 500 mg three times daily

- Selenium: 1,000 mcg daily

- B-complex: 100 mg daily

- Zinc citrate: 50 mg daily

- Vitamin E succinate: 800 IU daily

By April 26, 1999, most of the pain was gone, and he could run again with no pain. His appetite was good, and weight and energy normal. He still hoped to avoid surgery and planned to decide after his next CT scan and other examinations.

On December 29, 1999, he wrote that he had been busy in the fall and winter teaching at an American university and a local school. "Now that the holidays are upon us I have some time to catch up on life and emailing. My latest MRI (December 15th) again showed some good results and I will give you the tumor measurements since the first MRI in February of 1999.

	February	August	October	December
Length	13.0	12.0	11.5	11.0
Width	7.5	7.5	7.5	7.5
Height	12.0	11.0	10.5	9.0

(My note: volume was down from 1,170 to 743, a 36 percent decrease.)

"The tumor had taken a bit of a beating thanks largely to your suggested vitamin/mineral treatment, positive state of mind and a very nutritious diet. Considering the tumor is a three-dimensional object the shrinkage in volume has been considerable. Also a sarcoma specialist at the Cancer Clinic in Calgary has also suggested carrying on with the current treatment.

"I have also forwarded my current situation and results to the doctor in Toronto in two different emails but I have never received a response (specialist in pelvic oncology). I suppose he is not interested in complimentary or alternative treatment. Without our initial meeting I could very well be living with a fused hip.

Further I have also added some Chinese herbs to the treatment and any little pain that I had before seems to have abated. This was added in December after meeting with a Traditional Chinese Doctor (with a specialty in treating cancer) that I consulted with in Beijing, China."

In June 2003, he reported that the tumor, after a long period of quiescence, had started to shrink again.

Lymphoma

The number of patients surviving by years is shown below.

Survival Rate	1 Year	2 Years	3 Years
Orthomolecular Treatment—N 42	29	19	14
Standard Treatment—N 6	3	2	0

Case History: Patient #74

Patient #74 was born in 1947, and first seen in 1982. He was referred because of his severe depression. I started him on an antidepressant and on 1 gram of niacin three times daily and the same amount of vitamin C.

In June 1983, he was discovered to have a small cell diffuse lymphocyte lymphoma described as not curable. The clinic gave him three to six months. He was treated with surgery, irradiation, and chemotherapy, and I increased his vitamin C to 12 grams daily. By March 1984, he had a diffuse mass posteriorly on the left side of his chest, and he was given more radiation. By May, that cleared that mass, but by June, it had recurred as a para spinal mass separated from the previous mass. More chemotherapy followed, and more radiotherapy, but by then he had a left side effusion lymphomas infiltrate. By June 1984, more nodes were enlarged. More chemotherapy followed in July, but in August, he was found to have a persistent incurable malignant disease. By September 1984, he was symptom free and he refused any more treatment.

In January 1985, a large right pelvic mass was discovered, and he agreed to receive more radiation. This was his eighth recurrence. For a while he took 40 grams of vitamin C daily. When I asked him had he had any diarrhea, he said he had. He told me that he "sat on the can all day and read," and considering the alternative, he did not mind. By March 1986, he was well. His oncologist was not happy with his use of the orthomolecular program. He wrote in his file, "I can no longer feel an intra-abdominal mass. Unfortunately, he started on large doses of vitamin C and B vitamins prior to therapy and he was convinced that these are responsible for his good response rather than the chemotherapy." In mid 2002, his tumor markers suddenly began to increase. For several years, he had been taking very little vitamin C. He promptly increased his vitamin C to 40 grams per day, and one month later the markers were normal. As of October 2003, he was well, and symptom free.

Case History: Patient #573

Patient #573 was born in 1931, and first seen in 1994. He had suffered from duodenal ulcer with pain for many years, which responded to treatment each time it recurred. Early in 1994, the pain did not subside, and he was found to have a low-grade lymphoma around his stomach.

He was started on daily doses of 12 grams of ascorbic acid, 1.5 grams of niacinamide, 50 mg of B complex, 200 mcg of selenium, 50 mg of zinc citrate, 800 IU of vitamin E, and 300 mg of coenzyme Q_{10}. In June, a large mass and one-half of his stomach was resected. The tumor was more aggressive than had been expected. He was given chemotherapy for his large cell lymphoma, and he also arranged to take 50 to 100 grams intravenous vitamin C on three occasions. By May 1995, he was well.

In August 2002, he noted a lump in his abdominal wall. Needle aspiration showed a recurrence of a diffuse small cell lesion and he received more chemotherapy. By July, he had completed six chemotherapy sessions and his tumor had decreased to half its size, but pleural effusions had developed. Lymphatic fluid from his intestinal tract was emptying into his pleural cavity, the space within the chest that holds the lungs. He was admitted to the hospital, and each day for ten days, one liter of fluid was removed. He lost a lot of weight. He was offered more chemotherapy as palliative treatment.

Upon discharge from the hospital, he started to take 2 grams of curcumin (tumeric—an antioxidant

and powerful anticancer agent) three times daily reinforced with 5 mg of bioperin (an extract from black
pepper fruit) three times daily to improve the curcumin absorption. After another series of chemotherapy, his tumor disappeared, to the surprise of his
family doctor and his oncologist. By February 2003,
he was well again. He had regained his weight, and
felt better than he had in the previous fifteen years.
When he was last seen in October 2003, he remained
normal and enthusiastic.

Cancer of the Pancreas

Cancer of the pancreas is one of the deadliest forms
of cancer, and hardly any patients survive one year.
Every one of my control group died within one year
after I first saw them. By contrast, the treated group
did better; out of twenty-one, seven lived more than
one year, and three lived more than five years.

The number of patients surviving by years is
shown below.

Survival Rate	1 Year	2 Years	5 Years
Orthomolecular Treatment—N 21	7	5	3
Standard Treatment—N 14	0	0	0

CHAPTER 15

CANCER AND
SCHIZOPHRENIA

Ihave been working with the hypothesis that adrenochrome is involved as one of the main factors
in the cause of schizophrenia since 1952. Adrenochrome is an oxidation product
of adrenaline (epinephrine). All
of the catecholamines can be
oxidized in the same way, dopamine into dopachrome, for example. I described this hypothesis
and the hallucinogenic properties of adrenochrome in *The
Hallucinogens*, which I wrote with
Dr. Humphry Osmond.

Catecholamines
*Brain chemicals that
act as communication
carriers between nerves.
These include dopamine,
epinephrine (adrenaline),
and norepinephrine
(noradrenaline).*

Adrenochrome is also toxic to mitosis, the process
of cell division, so it appeared plausible that there
would be a natural antagonism between cancer
and schizophrenia if our hypothesis was correct.
Since cancer is the result of uncontrolled cell division,
it could not coexist with adrenochrome. If a patient
made too much adrenochrome due to extreme
amounts of adrenaline oxidation, he could develop
schizophrenia but not cancer, because the adrenochrome would inhibit cell division. If a patient did not
make enough adrenochrome, he could get cancer
but not schizophrenia, because there would not be
enough adrenochrome present to exert its hallucinogenic properties.

This was my hypothesis, and, in fact, that is what I
found. I have seen over 5,000 patients with schizophrenia and over 1,200 patients with cancer since
1955. Only ten of these patients had both cancer
and schizophrenia. Each recovered with professional
care, which included the type of treatment described

in this book. I have not seen one schizophrenic patient die from cancer. This clear antagonism between cancer and schizophrenia applies, but not to the same degree, to first order relatives of the patient. Here is what I found, Foster and Hoffer (2004):

	Number of Relatives	Relatives with Schizophrenia	Relatives with Cancer
Patients with Cancer— N 114	785	3	89
Patients with Schizophrenia— N 95	437	29	26

In Finland, a major study found that the incidence of cancer among schizophrenic patients was lower than it was in the general population. This confirms similar findings published in the literature.

My conclusion is that schizophrenia patients with cancer who receive the combination of standard and orthomolecular treatment methods will recover from both diseases. The decrease in incidence of cancer may be another factor that makes schizophrenia a genetic morphism, a disease that has survived in spite of major efforts for many years to prevent its reproduction. I suggest it is a genetic morphism with Huxley, Mayr, and Osmond (1964), and elaborate on this in Foster and Hoffer (2004). Schizophrenia may be evolving as a major defense against cancer. Horrobin (2001) reviewed the evidence for this, and postulates that the responsible gene or genes are spreading into the entire population.

For many years, investigators have been searching desperately for chemicals or drugs, whether natural or not, that might be valuable in treating cancer, but very little time and money has been spent looking for compounds normally made in the body that might play a role. We really must have clues about where to look. Without a clue, it is impossible to guess. The inverse association between schizophrenia and cancer provides such a clue. I really think it is vital for re-search scientists to look at the role played by the oxidized derivatives of adrenaline, such as adreno-chrome. They inhibit the growth of rapidly dividing cells.

CONCLUSION

The results of orthomolecular treatments have been studied by many respected scientists. These studies have included years of clinical research, and close follow-up of patients who have used traditional medical treatment methods only, and those who have followed a combination treatment plan including both orthomolecular and traditional treatments. Their conclusions give added hope to patients diagnosed with cancer.

In spite of the overwhelming evidence to the contrary, many practitioners of traditional medicine, including oncologists, radiologists, and others involved in cancer treatment, still discount the validity of orthomolecular treatments. Years of observations and results, provided by well-known and respected researchers, are rejected as anecdotal, and there is concern that supplementation could affect the standard course of treatment. This has not proved to be true in practice; indeed, orthomolecular treatments have been shown to improve the outcome of standard treatments such as radiation. This rejection is also based on the claim that there is a lack of large, standard, traditional clinical trials, which are difficult to fund and perform outside of large institutions, but it is coming, as patients and their families begin to demand this added course of treatment. It is interesting to note that such trials are, at the current time, often funded by large drug companies. The nutrients used in orthomolecular supplementation are freely available and do not require expensive patents and prescriptions.

It is important for your doctor to understand that orthomolecular treatment is not intended to replace standard cancer treatment, but to supplement it as part of a full treatment program. It will not negatively impact any traditional treatments. There is clear evidence that supports the hypothesis that adding nutrients to the standard treatment of cancer is very beneficial to patients. Our in-the-field practical experience with cancer patients shows that the supplementation presented in this book to be a plausible course of treatment for any cancer patient. It is true that the increased response rate cannot be estimated from just this series of patients. Such a conclusion will have to await the outcome of large-scale prospective randomized controlled studies. However, the treatment will do no harm, and can have a positive effect on the health and longevity of the patient. It only seems logical that until the outcome of the controlled trials is available, patients ought to be given the potential benefit and added hope that orthomolecular treatment can provide.

SELECTED
REFERENCES

Ames, BN, Elson-Schwab I, Silver, EA. High-dose vitamin therapy stimulates variant enzymes with decreased coenzymes binding affinity (increased K_m): relevance to genetic disease and polymorphisms[1-3]. *American Journal of Clinical Nutrition,* 2002;75:616–58.

Burke, KE. Oral and topical L-selenomethionine protection from ultraviolet-induced sunburn, tanning and skin cancer. *Journal of Orthomolecular Medicine,* 1992;7:83–94.

Burke, KE, Combs, GF, Jr, Gross, EG, et al. The effects of topical and oral L-selenomethionine on pigmentation and skin cancer induced by ultraviolet irradiation. *Nutrition and Cancer,* 1992;17:123–37.

Cancer Prevention Coalition. *Stop Cancer Before it starts. The Campaign on How to Win the Losing War Against Cancer.* Chicago, IL, University of Illinois at Chicago, School of Pubic Health.

Canner, PL, Berge, KG, Wenger, NK, et al. Fifteen year mortality coronary drug project; Patients long term benefit with niacin. *American College of Cardiology,* 1986;8:1245–1255.

Drisko, AD, Hapman, J, Hunter, VJ. The use of antioxidants with first-line chemotherapy in two cases of ovarian cancer. *Journal of the American College of Nutrition,* 2003;22: 118–123.

Foster, HD. *Health, Disease and The Environment.* CRC Press, Boca Raton, FL, 1992.

Foster, HD. *What really causes AIDS.* Trafford Publishers, Victoria, BC. 2002.

Foster, HD, Hoffer, A. *Schizophrenia and Cancer: The Adrenochrome Balanced Morphism. Medical Hypotheses.* In Press, 2004; 62:415–419.

Gerson, M. Dietary considerations in malignant neoplastic disease: a prelimary report. *The Review of Gastroenterology,* 1945;12:419–425.

Gerson, M. Effects of a combined dietary regime on patients with malignant tumors. *Experimental Medicine and Surgery,* 1949;7:299–317.

Gignac, MA. Antioxidants and Chemotherapy. What You

Need to Know Before Following Dr. Labriola's Advice. *Townsend Letter for Doctors and Patients,* Feb/March 2000:88–89.

Goodman, S. *Nutrition and cancer: state of the art.* Bristol, UK: Positive Health Publications, 1998.

Heaney, RP. Long-latency deficiency disease: insights from calcium and vitamin D. *American Journal of Clinical Nutrition,* 2003;78:912–919.

Hoffer, A. Orthomolecular Oncology. In, *Adjuvant Nutrition in Cancer Treatment,* Quillin, P, Williams, RM, editors. 1992 Symposium Proceedings. Arlington Heights, IL: Cancer Treatment Research Foundation, 1994;331–362.

Hoffer, A. *Hoffer's Laws of Natural Nutrition: A Guide to Eating Well for Pure Health.* Kingston, ON: Quarry Press, 1996.

Hoffer, A., Pauling, L. *Vitamin C and Cancer: Discovery, Recovery, Controversy.* Kingston, ON: Quarry Press, 2000.

Hoffer, A, Pauling, L. Hardin Jones biostatistical analysis of mortality data for cohorts of cancer patients with a large fraction surviving at the termination of the study and a comparison of survival times of cancer patients receiving large regular oral doses of vitamin C and other nutrients with similar patients not receiving those doses. *Journal of Orthomolecular Medicine,* 5:143–154,1990. Reprinted in: Cameron, E, Pauling, L, *Cancer and Vitamin C,* updated and expanded. Philadelphia, PA: Camino Books, 1993.

Hoffer, A. Antioxidant Nutrients and Cancer. *Journal of Orthomolecular Medicine,* 2000;193–200.

Hoffer, LJ. Nutrients as biologic response modifiers. In, *Adjuvant Nutrition in Cancer Treatment.* Quillin, P, Williams, RM, editors. Arlington Heights, IL. Cancer Treatment Research Foundation. 1993;55–79.

Hoffer, LJ. Vitamin C: Case History of an Alternative Cancer Therapy. *Journal of Orthomolecular Medicine,* 2000;15:181–188.

Hoffer, LJ, Tamayo, C, Richardson, MA. Vitamin C as Cancer Therapy: An Overview. *Journal of Orthomolecular Medicine,* 2000;15:175–180.

Horrobin, D. *Humanity.* London: Bantam Press, 2001.

Huxley, J, Mayr, E, Osmond, H, Hoffer, A. Schizophrenia as a genetic morphism. *Nature,* 1964:204:220–221.

Jacobson, M, Jacobson, E. *Niacin, nutrition, ADP-ribosylation and cancer. The 8th International Symposium on ADP-Ribosylation,* Fort Worth, TX: Texas College of Osteopathic Medicine, 1987.

Knekt, P, Aromaa, A, Maatela, J, et al. Vitamin E and cancer prevention. *American Journal of Clinical Nutrition*, 1991; 53:283S-286S.

Labriola, D, Livingston, R. Possible interactions between dietary antioxidants and chemotherapy. *Oncology*, 1999;13: 1003–1008.

Labriola, D, Livingston, R. Editorial. *Townsend Letter for Doctors and Patients*, November 1999.

Lawson, S. On Vitamin C. *Journal of Orthomolecular Medicine*, 2003;18:173–186.

Moss, RW. *Questioning Chemotherapy*. Equinox Press Inc., Brooklyn, New York, 1995.

Moss, RW. *Antioxidants Against Cancer*. Equinox Press Inc., Brooklyn, New York, 2000.

Prasad, KN, Kumar, A, Kochupillai, V, et al. High doses of multiple antioxidant vitamins: essential ingredients in improving the efficacy of standard cancer therapy. *Journal of the American College of Nutrition*, 1999;18:13–25.

Rampersaud, GC, Bailey, LB, Kauwell, PA. Relationship of folate to colorectal and cervical cancer: review and recommendations for practitioners. *Journal of the American Dietetic Association*, 2002;102:1273–1281.

Reilly, P. Labriola's Editorial on Antioxidants and Chemotherapy, *Townsend Letter for Doctors and Patients*, Feb/Mar 2000;90–91.

Riordan, NH, Riordan, HD, Casciari, JP. Clinical and experimental experiences with intravenous vitamin C. *Journal of Orthomolecular Medicine*, 2000;15:201–213.

Smithells, RW, Sheppard, S, Wild, J, et al. Prevention of neural tube defect recurrence in Yorkshire: final report. *Lancet*, 1989; II:498–499.

Journal of Orthomolecular Medicine Special Issue, 2003;18: 123–219. Available from International Schizophrenia Foundation. e-mail: center@orthomed.org; website: www.orthomed.org

Tamayo, C, Richardson, MA. Vitamin C as a cancer treatment: state of the science and recommendations for research. *Alternative Therapies*, 2003;9:94–102.

Wahrendorf, J, Munoz, N, Lu, JB. Blood, retinal and zinc riboflavin status in relation to precancerous lesions of the oesophagus: findings from a vitamin intervention trial in the Peoples Republic of China. *Cancer Research*, 1988;48:2280–3.

Yu, S, Mai, B, Xiao, P, et al. Intervention trial with selenium for the prevention of lung cancer among tin miners in Yunnan, China. a pilot study. *Biological Trace Element Research*, 1990;24:105–108.

OTHER BOOKS
AND RESOURCES

Cameron, E, Pauling, L, *Cancer and Vitamin C,* updated and expanded. Philadelphia, PA: Camino Books, 1993.

Cancer Prevention Coalition. *Stop Cancer Before It Starts. The Campaign on How to Win the Losing War Against Cancer.* University of Illinois at Chicago, School of Pubic Health, Chicago, IL. Free download www.preventcancer. com

Cousins, N. *Anatomy of an Illness as Perceived by the Patient.* Norton, 1979.

Foster, HD. *What Really Causes AIDS.* Trafford Publishers, Victoria, BC. 2002. Free download www.hdfoster.com

Hoffer, A. *Hoffer's Laws of Natural Nutrition: A Guide to Eating Well for Pure Health.* Kingston, ON: Quarry Press, 1996.

Hoffer, A, Pauling, L. *Vitamin C and Cancer: Discovery, Recovery, Controversy.* Kingston, ON: Quarry Press, 2000.

GreatLife Magazine
Consumer magazine with articles on vitamins, minerals, herbs, and foods.
Available for free at many health and natural food stores.

Let's Live Magazine
Consumer magazine with emphasis on the health benefits of vitamins, minerals, and herbs.

Customer service:
1-800-676-4333
P.O. Box 74908
Los Angeles, CA 90004
Subscriptions: 12 issues per year, $19.95 in the U.S.; $31.95 outside the U.S.

Physical Magazine

Magazine oriented to bodybuilders and other serious athletes.

Customer service:
1-800-676-4333
P.O. Box 74908
Los Angeles, CA 90004

Subscriptions: 12 issues per year, $19.95 in the U.S.;
$31.95 outside the U.S.

The Nutrition Reporter™ newsletter

Monthly newsletter that summarizes recent medical research on vitamins, minerals, and herbs.

Customer service:
P.O. Box 30246
Tucson, AZ 85751-0246
e-mail: jack@thenutritionreporter.com
www.nutritionreporter.com

Subscriptions: 12 issues per year, $26 in the U.S.;
$32 U.S. or $48 CNC for Canada; $38 for other
countries.

INDEX

Printed in the USA
CPSIA information can be obtained
at www.ICGtesting.com
ISHW012008140824
68134JS00004B/63